Praise for Enlightened Eating and Caroline:

"This is more than a cookbook, or a collection of amazing recipes with thought-provoking quotes. It's a loving, inspiring gift. Caroline's spirit shines through on every page."
SANDRA ENTWISTLE

"I've had the pleasure and honour of knowing Caroline for many years now. The sincere and absolute commitment she has to being an example of aliveness and total health is an inspiration to us all. How fortunate we are that the collaboration of her creative ideas and discoveries are made available in this treasure-filled book. It will certainly nourish you, body, mind, heart and soul."
JILL HEWLETT, SPEAKER, TV HOST, PERSONAL AND GROUP LEADER

"In Enlightened Eating, as with her cooking classes, Caroline chooses the most effective combinations of fresh, healthy ingredients for easy-to-follow, foolproof recipes with consistently delicious results. You'll find a wide variety of dishes in this book, some unusual and some a bit exotic, yet always accessible to the home cook. And as I do, you'll want to make many of these well-tested recipes into frequently enjoyed staples in your own kitchen."
RICKI HELLER, OWNER, BAKE IT HEALTHY, INC. AND RICKI'S KITCHEN COOKING CLASSES

"Caroline's approach is heartfelt and honest with delicious results. Her practical approach to vegetarian and raw food is contagious and her recipes can be easily replicated — no fuss required!"
EVELYNE GHARIBIAN, HEARTYCATERING.COM

"I have been preparing meals from Enlightened Eating for seven years now and it has completely transformed the way my husband and I eat. It has been our guide from the beginning to making healthy choices for our two children who are now 6 and 4. Thanks to Caroline they know nothing other than healthy and delicious food. Not only has this book transformed the way I view nutrition but it has been both a spiritual and emotional awakening. This is the only cookbook I use or could ever recommend."
SHANNON HARLOW

"Enlightened Eating has allowed my family and friends to make better health choices. Caroline's message is clear and practical with fantastic, simple recipes. We can all make healthy conscious eating a part of our lives after reading this book."
LORI PEARSON

"Enlightened Eating is like Caroline herself: full of grace and wisdom. A gentle and practical approach to nourishing our body/mind/spirit through our food. It contains healthy cooked and raw food choices, which distinguishes it from nearly any other recipe book out there. I use it to feed my family and highly recommend it to clients and friends."
SHANNON LEONNE, LIFE-COACH, AUTHOR AND SPEAKER

"Delicious, simple, and healthy, the recipes in Enlightened Eating are true extensions of Caroline's love for holistic healing through natural, whole foods. May your copy of Enlightened Eating be as used (crinkled and stained) as mine!"
SUSAN BAKER,
REGISTERED HOLISTIC NUTRITIONIST AND TEACHER AT THE CANADIAN SCHOOL OF NATURAL NUTRITION

"Whenever we cook for others,
we are making a statement to them.
If what we prepare and present
to our family and guests
is attractive, tasty, and health-supporting,
we are saying that we want them to be well and happy,
to feel nurtured and strengthened.
When we offer cuisine that is made of
whole and natural ingredients,
we are saying that we want them
to have all the energy they need
in order to make every aspect of their lives richer.
We are saying that we honor them."

JOHN ROBBINS, IN MAY ALL BE FED

Enlightened Eating

Nourishment for Body and Soul

BY CAROLINE MARIE DUPONT

"And I saw a new Heaven and a new Earth...
I heard a voice saying
there shall be no more death,
neither sorrow, nor crying,
for the former things are passed away."

ESSENE BOOK OF REVELATIONS

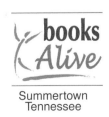

books
Alive

Summertown
Tennessee

COVER ART BY CÉSAN D'ORNELLAS LEVINE
"As an artist, I am drawn away from a rendering of the outer, towards an expression of the inner life, light and love that enlivens us."

Césan's expressive abstracts are painted on canvas using a wide array of acrylic paints and media. She is known for courageous use of colour, richly layered application and generous textural work. Césan exhibits and sells her work through galleries, special venues, private collectors and by commission. Visit www.cesan.ca for more information and to view more work.

Copyright © 2006 by Caroline Marie Dupont

Published in the United States by
Books Alive
P.O. Box 99
Summertown, TN 38483
1-888-260-8458

www.bookpubco.com

Printed in Canada
ISBN 978-1-55312-042-1

14 13 12 11 10 09   7 6 5 4 3 2

Edited by Barb Payne
Designed by Cathy Russell
Author photo by Celine Saki

All rights reserved. No portion of this book may be reproduced by any means whatsoever, except for brief quotations in reviews, without written permission from the publisher.

The Library of Congress has already cataloged an earlier printing under the publisher name "Alive Books" as follows:
Dupont, Caroline Marie.
 Enlightened eating : nourishment for body and soul / By Caroline Marie Dupont.
    p. cm.
 Includes index.
 ISBN 978-1-55312-042-1
 1. Cookery (Natural foods) 2. Meditation. I. Title.
 TX741.D85 2007
 641.5'63--dc22   2007016857

We are a member of Green Press Initiative. We chose to print this title on paper with postconsumer recycled content and processed chlorine free, which saved the following natural resources:

7 trees	5 million BTU of total energy	
340 pounds of solid waste	637 pounds of greenhouse gases	
2,647 gallons of water		

For more information visit: www.greenpressinitiative.org. Savings calculations from the Environmental Defense Paper Calculator at www.edf.org/papercalculator.

I lovingly dedicate this book to my children,
Jérémie and Jacqueline,
and to the child in each one of us
who naturally lives guided by the heart.

Acknowledgments

My life has been blessed by support from a seemingly infinite number of sources. I have been inspired by many pioneers of natural health and living who, through their writings and lectures, have passed on to me their passion and enthusiasm for their life's work and their commitment to serving humanity by helping people live their lives to the fullest.

I WOULD LIKE TO THANK:

My family, friends, and students for encouraging and supporting me in my dreams and aspirations.

My mother, Gisèle, for giving me my first experiences in the kitchen and, through your nourishment, nurturing my own ability to care about and honour people through food.

My father, John, for your steadfastness and dedication to all your children.

Jérémie and Jacqueline, for inspiring me from our very first encounters, being such shining examples of soulful living and health, and for eating and enjoying the food that we share together!

Robert Warren, for your love and support throughout this process, and for the deep lessons. I will forever be grateful for the gifts that you shared, the work that we have done together–I have been nourished more than I can express in words.

My colleagues at the Canadian School of Natural Nutrition: Danielle Perrault, for having faith in me and giving me the opportunity to teach when the school was taking it's first steps and to Lisa Tsakos for helping to pave the way; CSNN managers Leslie Gould, Vivian Lee, Carolyn Steiss and Pat Ward, and all of the instructors for embarking with me on this most fulfilling task of educating human beings about the profound importance of eating well.

The students, who I have had the pleasure to teach and to learn from, for your faith in me as a teacher, sharing of yourselves, and helping me learn, through teaching, what I strive to embody.

Cathy Russell, for your encouragement, tireless work, keen eye and loving contributions to this project.

Barb Payne, for your attention to the most minute details and your genuine care in the editing process.

Césan d'Ornellas Levine, for your generous spirit and brilliant artwork.

Nancy Battaglia, Cathy Bell, Tari Lee Cornish, Carole Craig, Kim Cross, Francine Dupont, Lee Dupont, Marianne Dupont, Arbor Eichmann, Evelyne Gharibian, Linda Gilbert, Deb Griffith, Shannon Harlow, Jill Hewlett, Carolyn Molnar, Gloria Oduardi, Janet Osborne, Maie Paluka, Deb Peterson, Andrea Roth, Suzie Saint Yves, Julia Smith, Kathy Stapleton, Ginette Veugelers, Deborah Whipple, and all the many other special women in my life, for your beauty and your courage, and for reminding me of what it is to be a woman in these times.

Contents

Blessed with this food and this life,
We offer thanks.
Thanks to the Earth, to the Sun, to the Moon, to the Stars;
Thanks to the streams of water, to the pools, to the springs,
to the lakes, to the oceans;
Thanks to the mountains, to the forests,
to the meadows, to the valleys;
Thanks to the grasses, to the vegetables, to the fruit,
to the seeds, to the medicinal herbs;
Thanks to the wind, to the clouds, to the rain;
Thanks to the Great One at the source of all things,
Who is the giver of breath and of health and of life.
May this meal be taken in gratitude.
May our lives be lived in gratitude.

FROM MAY ALL BE FED BY JOHN ROBBINS

Foreword

There has been a tremendous change in people's attitudes towards food and nutrition in the past ten years.

Expert advice is available everywhere, through magazine articles, books, internet, and every other means of communication. The average consumer is well on his or her way to becoming better educated and more knowledgeable as to what to eat.

When even corporate owners of fast food chains recognize the need to include healthy foods choices on their menus in order to hang on to their market, it is easy to see that good progress is being made.

This progress can be credited to the quickening of a global awareness regarding the role of nutrition in our lives. It is, however, only the tip of the iceberg. Self-responsibility quickly follows the realization of the importance of healthy foods to human health. This, in turn, opens the way to a better comprehension of the concept of body-mind-spirit. Feeding the body properly feeds the Mind and Soul as well.

Most of us are still relatively new to this advanced concept of nutrition. Some, by the gift of an uncommon wisdom, have already made giant steps in that direction. The author of this book, Caroline Marie Dupont, is one of those gifted people. She not only understands intimately the relationship between what we eat and who we are, but she applies this knowledge to her own life and shares it generously with all who will listen.

It is predictable that, in the next decade, we will see a strong movement towards bettering the quality and safety of our food chain. This will bring us closer to Nature, the Great Provider. It will direct our attention to our own communities as the ideal source of quality foods and, hopefully, we will see a resurgence of interest in our own farming environment and local organic enterprises.

The way is simple really, and we can confidently follow Caroline as she leads us to better health.

Danielle Perrault, RHN
Director, Canadian School of Natural Nutrition
March 5th, 2006

Create in me a pure heart
O my God,
and renew a tranquil conscience within me
O my hope.
Through the spirit of power confirm Thou me in Thy cause
O my best beloved,
And by the light of thy glory reveal unto me Thy path
O Thou the goal of my desire.
By the power of Thy transcendent might lift me up
unto the heaven of Thy holiness
O source of my being,
And by the breezes of Thine eternity gladden me
O Thou who art my God.
Let Thine everlasting melodies breathe tranquility on me
O my companion,
And let the riches of Thine ancient countenance
deliver me from all except Thee
O my master.
And let the tidings of the revelation
of Thine incorruptible essence gladden me
O Thou who art the most manifest of the manifest
and the most hidden of the hidden.

BAHA'I PRAYER

Introduction: The Heart's Way to Health

Food... we make choices every day that affect, perhaps more than anything else, our looks, health, energy level, longevity, mood, and state of mind. Day after day we continue struggling to make the right choices, we read new health and nutrition books, we try new diets, we buy new supplements, and yet true health still eludes us. What is the answer?

This book is my current contribution to the answer, but it's more than just giving the answer—it's a book about possibilities. It has come from a lifetime of study and application of nutritional, health, and spiritual principles. So far, I have discovered that the solution is both very simple and very complex. Simple because the answers have been lying inside each one of us forever—nature has been providing us with the proper foods since the beginning of time, and we do have the ability to access the intuition to consistently choose the most health-supporting foods for ourselves and our families. Complex because we have strayed so far—we are a society that looks for shortcuts, and we are painfully alienated from the natural world and from an intimate relationship with our physical, emotional, and spiritual bodies.

In writing this book, my intention is to provide inspirational and practical information that will guide you towards a greater understanding of your relationship with food—so that you can effortlessly select and prepare foods that are healthy and healing for you and your loved ones. I have come to understand, through my experience in the health field, that lasting change must come from the deeper levels of our being. Although important, it is not enough to simply change habits. We need to develop a deeper understanding of how our food choices influence our physical, mental, emotional, and spiritual health. Our food choices directly affect our energy fields, which are the blueprints for our physical bodies. Eating food is how we take in and transform the energies of the universe—energies which have been absorbed and stored by each vegetable, leaf, seed, nut, and fruit, and released as a gift from Nature to us when we consume them. I believe that, once we fully understand not only the importance and intimacy of our relationship with our environment, but also how delicate that relationship is, making correct health-supporting choices becomes effortless, joyful, and satisfying.

We must acknowledge that all diseases can be prevented, improved, or cured through food. Right diet may not always be enough, but few diseases can be alleviated without it. Food enables us to free the natural wisdom in each of our bodies—the wisdom that says that this body knows how to be healthy and longs to be healthy. And ultimately, through health we will claim our God given right for joy, abundance, and fulfillment.

On a Personal Note: One Person's Journey

This book represents a 17-year journey into the compelling and powerful world of nutrition. In it you will find gleanings from vegetarianism, veganism, macrobiotics, Ayurveda, and live foods philosophies. However, as much as vegetarian philosophies and recipes make up a large part of these writings, my hope is that it will appeal to anyone who is interested in health no matter what that means for them at this time in their life. There is no longer any doubt, based on scientific research and long-term observation of various populations, that we could all benefit from at least decreasing our intake of animal products. Also, woven into this book are approaches to human change—the psychology of transformation fascinates me and stems from my longing to reach and help as many beings as possible who are ready to embrace healthy living through nutrition. It represents my own observations through the years of feeding my family and friends, teaching nutrition and holistic health, embracing universal and natural principles, and holding ongoing cooking and food preparation classes in my home.

And so it is a book dedicated to each of our own journeys towards a nutritional approach that works in our lives: that makes us vibrant, that makes best use of our time, that considers our full lives and our need to please and nourish our families, and mostly recognizes and honours our varying paths to the common goals of wholeness, health, and peace.

There are some things that I wonder about and simultaneously know at the core of my being—when we eat fake foods we become less authentic; when our foods are fractioned we become less centered; when we eat chemical residues that are designed to kill life, we die a little; when we eat food that is grown or raised with an element of human or animal suffering, we become hardened to our natural compassion for all life; when we choose foods only because of speed and convenience, we perpetuate the madness that rules our days.

And so when we begin to make food choices that affirm health, we say yes to all that is good. I cannot help but believe that, not only would our hospitals no longer be bursting at the seams, but that there would be less crime and less disharmony in our societies, our families, and within ourselves. The effects of food on our physical and psycho-spiritual health are immense. I look forward to the day when the people of the world appreciate food for the healer that it is. There are very few healing modalities that can affect us so constantly and powerfully. Every meal is an affirmation of our desire to be more alive and more energized physically, mentally, emotionally, and spiritually.

It is well-known that natural, alive, high-quality foods clearly create healthier physical bodies. Virtually every disorder can be prevented, improved, or healed through food. You will enjoy better energy, endurance, strength, skin quality, and brighter eyes. You will effortlessly arrive at a healthy weight. Once you begin to consume higher quality foods, you will also notice changes in your mental state—a greater ability to focus, more positive thinking, a calmer mind, more peace, and a more open mind. Emotionally, you will begin to be more honest with yourself and others about your feelings; you will begin to be able to let emotions flow through you more easily; and there will be fewer fluctuations in your emotional state. There will be an underlying level of joy regardless of what else is happening in your life at the time. When you become clearer and cleaner physically, mentally, and emotionally, you will begin to connect more deeply with the part of you that has been called true self, core, inner light, spirit, or soul. Your inner light is able to shine more freely through a clear body and mind.

Food has been such a blessing in my life—it has brought me back to life, to my connection with the Earth, to my wholeness, to my multi-dimensionality, to my belonging to the web.

Nutrition is truly a healing art.

There are a few recollections of my early life that stand out as I reflect on how I came to be where I am today. One very clear picture that stands out in my mind is a poster of Desiderata that I taped on my bedroom closet door and memorized at 10-years-old: "Go placidly among the noise and the haste and remember what peace there may be in silence..." Two books also remain in my heart's memory: Jonathan Livingston Seagull by Richard Bach and The Story of Tom Dooley, an American doctor working as a missionary in China. Jonathan Livingston Seagull gave me a longing for freedom, peace, and authenticity. I think the Tom Dooley book reminded me of a purpose etched in my soul long ago to bring peace to others through physical and spiritual healing. The clearest longing that I recall as a feeling from my childhood was for a closeness to God and for the fullness and joy of fulfilling my life's purpose.

As a teenager all of this seemed to go dormant as I kept busy with school, piano, ballet, part-time jobs, and friends. I married my high school sweetheart at 22, and followed him to Chicago where he played hockey for the Chicago Blackhawks.

The birth of my first child at 27 marked the beginning of my awakening. It seems as though I transformed from one day to the next. Before Jérémie was born I was somewhat like a robot, programmed to think and act in certain ways that seemed safe but were not a true reflection of me. Looking back, I can see that I was pretty hardened to myself and others. I fell in love with Jérémie instantly and it lit a fire in me that began to melt whatever it was that separated me from my heart. I cried almost every time I held him for the first couple of weeks—when I felt the love that opened my heart, I invariably felt the ache of pain that had lodged itself in me from days and lives gone by. It was so amazing that this sweet, pink, little bundle could be more powerful than anything I had ever encountered. He touched me. I remember when he was 3-days-old, walking through the halls of the hospital not wanting to return him to the nursery, and our eyes locked for the first time—what I saw was wisdom and love and purity, and recognition. And so this was the beginning of my transformation—within a year, I went from being mainstream to becoming a vegetarian, an environmentalist, and a natural health advocate.

Jérémie's birth changed my view of the world in several ways. I discovered the true power of deep love—here was this babe who transformed me without a single word, just by being his brilliant little self. By opening up my heart to him, I began to open my heart to my true self. Also, I recognized that the ability to change is in all of us. If I could transform—asleep being that I was—then anyone could. This has served me as a teacher because I see the potential for growth in everyone and have faith in the power of every being's soul to dislodge unconscious behaviour. And I learned that what ignites the soul is unconditional love. I am so fortunate to have received that from Jérémie and later from my sweet Jacqueline from our very first encounters.

As I was nursing Jérémie, I began to plan for the day when I would eventually feed him solid foods. I took advantage of my time at home with him to read all that I could about various nutritional approaches. Diet for A New America, by John Robbins, is a brilliant and courageous book on vegetarianism as an approach to a more compassionate, healthy, and environmentally-conscious society. John was the only heir to the Baskin Robbins ice cream empire, and at 21 decided to leave and seek out his own path. I cried, was inspired, educated, reborn, moved, and ultimately transformed. There was no turning back.

In less than two weeks, my household became vegetarian. Although I was excited about our new direction, having been raised on a Four Food Groups approach to nutrition made it challenging at first. There were family and friends to confess to, concerns about our children's health to address, and of course the new repertoire of foods to prepare. It was daunting at first. Because we made the change so fast, and at the time we were cutting out dairy and eggs as well, every meal was a challenge. I would look in the fridge and wonder, "What am I going to make with these vegetables tonight?" Eventually, thanks to my then husband's support, to magazines like Vegetarian Times, and some good cookbooks and friendships that came our way, I began to get the hang of the vegetarian lifestyle. Except for a few flops, the variety of new foods and flavours that we were introduced to delighted us. I continued to read and educate myself in order to stay on track—food and nutrition had become a new passion, eventually leading me to become a Holistic Nutritionist and teach for the Canadian School of Natural Nutrition.

The dietary changes initiated shifts in virtually every other area of my life. I eventually achieved a Black Belt in the Nia Technique (a holistic movement form), became a student of yoga, and embarked on a journey to explore the psycho-spiritual aspects of my being. In the process, I have experienced, studied, and practiced various energy therapies that I now incorporate into my holistic health practice. I have rediscovered the freedom and joy of dancing, singing, pottery, drumming, gardening, growing some of our food, sustainable living, spending time in nature, and a disciplined spiritual practice. I am becoming more comfortable living in the magic of the unknown and look forward to a life of awakenings, synchronicities, laughter, service, and love.

"I wake sweet joy in dens of sorrow and I plant a smile in forests of affliction and wake the bubbling springs of life in regions of dark death." WILLIAM BLAKE

Enlightened Eating: A Self-Realization Diet

"We are all part of the One Spirit. When you experience the true meaning of religion, which is to know God, you will realize that He is your Self, and that He exists equally and impartially in all beings." PARAMAHANSA YOGANANDA

When I first began to explore diet and nutrition my goal was physical health. As an exercise physiologist and fitness instructor, I had reaped the rewards of a physically active lifestyle. Nutrition was to be the next piece of the health puzzle. In our shift to a vegetarian whole foods diet, we received many benefits such as increased energy, better digestion and elimination, and improved health in general. However, other unexpected transformations occurred for me—I connected with a deep longing for meaning and authenticity in my life. I seemed to be more aware, more alive, more curious about who I was and how I could fulfill my purpose here. In a manner of speaking, you could say that I reconnected with my soul. The more I felt and learned, the more this journey to my own soul and back to Source became the most important direction in my life.

I have come to believe that nutrition plays a very large part in the awakening of consciousness.

Self-realization is a term most commonly used in Eastern philosophies to define the ultimate goal to know our Self and to manifest the Divine within ourselves with perfect clarity. We use this state of being to transform our entire existence: our physical bodies, our minds, our work and service, and our relationship with others and the world around us.

Although most of us are aware of the body as a physical entity that can be experienced through the senses, the spiritual or energy body is in many ways far more real than our flesh and bones. What is the energy body? It has been called Prana, Chi, Astral Light, aura, electromagnetic field ... and mystics have been describing it and its properties for thousands of years. It is only in the last century that scientists have been able to measure and photograph it using instruments and specialized photography such as Kirlian. The following are some of the principles of the Universal Energy Field (the Human Energy Field is a component of it and is governed by the same principles)—later, I will relate this to food choices.

First, everything has an energy field, both animate and inanimate objects—a flower, a rock, a pen, this book, an apple, a bottle, a dog. Thoughts and emotions affect the universal energy field. Some people naturally have (or have developed) the ability to see, feel, sense, hear, and even smell energy fields.

Second, the energy field connects objects to one another through space and knows nothing of time. So, when you think of someone across the ocean and they call you shortly after, your thoughts, being energy, traveled and were received by someone who is receptive to them.

Third, the universal energy field follows the laws of harmonic inductance. Harmonic inductance is what happens when you strike a tuning fork and its vibration will start another silent fork resonating. In other words, we are affected by all of the various energy fields that we expose ourselves to. Say you meet with a friend for a chat. You are in a good mood, she is feeling miserable. What will happen at the end of your time together? Either your mood will slide down as result of her low vibration or her mood will come up as a result of your high vibration. Who wins this battle of the energy fields? The strongest vibration of course. So, if your good mood is a little precarious you will likely lose. The stronger your vibration, the less likely that you will be affected by others' energy fields. We have all experienced this.

So, if we are in fact affected by all of the energy fields that we expose ourselves to, it behooves us to strengthen our own field by surrounding ourselves with as much high vibration as possible in the form of positive supportive relationships, beauty in our homes and workplaces, uplifting music, peaceful surroundings, nature and objects from nature, etc.—and high quality food, of course. More about that shortly. The most powerful approach to strengthening our energy fields is a consistent spiritual practice, whatever that means to you. It could be a combination of prayer, meditation, breathwork, movement like yoga postures or dance, devotional activities, inspirational reading, service to others, church, connection with nature, etc.

Another interesting property of the universal energy field that follows from harmonic inductance is that objects take on the vibration of their owner or of any energy that they have come in contact with. This is how psychics pick up information on missing people from, for example, their hair brushes. This has repercussions when you purchase any object, especially second-hand objects like cars, clothes, jewelry, or even homes. There are many rituals, like smudging, that can be performed to clear the field.

Getting back to food though, if we are in fact energy fields and we want to hold as high a vibration as possible, and we are taking food into our bodies on an ongoing basis, it makes sense to choose food with a high vibration. Lettuce lovingly grown in your grandmother's garden and eaten fresh has a higher vibration than lettuce raised on a huge farm that sat under fluorescent lights in a large grocery store for a few days. This is aside from the obvious nutritional superiority. Which one would you choose? A tomato grown by an organic farmer who has a deep respect for the earth and a sincere concern for human health has a higher vibration (and a better taste I might add) than the tomato genetically-engineered to be a certain size and shape and to last longer on the shelves of the supermarket. Which one would you choose? A chicken raised free and allowed to peck at the earth in sunlight has a higher vibration than the chicken raised in the miserable conditions of factory farms today: caged, cramped, no natural light, no respect for basic instincts, driven mad. Do you understand the difference? Which egg would you choose? Have you ever had a meal prepared by someone in a terrible mood? Can you feel the energy in the food? Much of the flavour and enjoyment of a delicious dish comes from the positive energy of the person who prepares it.

The path to self-realization is an ongoing refinement, clearing, expansion, and brightening of our own human energy field. A clear energy field is bright, expanded, energized, and free-flowing.

Most people's energy fields are not clear. When perceived by the higher senses, they are found to have blocks, to be contracted, to have cloudy areas where energy is not flowing freely—this will eventually manifest as physical disease. As long as our energy fields are not clear, our inner light cannot shine through and we will continue to struggle in many or all aspects of our lives.

So the first thing to realize from all of this is that at our deepest level in the core of our being we are already perfect, bright, peaceful, and healthy. The Light is there but, like a lamp whose glass shade is covered with dust and soot, the light is dimmed. We can clean the shade in two ways. One, by cleaning it from the outside— metaphorically speaking, this is the process of looking at mental and emotional patterns that have put the layers of soot and dust there in the first place. Two, we can intensify our Light by connecting directly to our two sources: Heaven and Earth. Daily and moment-to-moment we care for both our spirit and our body. Like a battery, and any energy field, we need to be plugged into both the positive (Heaven, electric) and negative (Earth, magnetic) poles to activate electromagnetic energy flow. As the Light's intensity increases in this way, it automatically burns off the soot and dust through its heat and inherent energy. So strengthen your inner Light by plugging into your two primary sources: connect to your spiritual body throughout your days in whatever ways feel real for you AND take infinite care of your physical body in all of the ways that you know of and can incorporate into your life on a regular basis.

To be self-realized is to be in a state of clear-being. We have dissolved our energy blocks through awareness, inner work, and consistent care of the soul and the body. We can then go out into the world to bring much needed love, service and peace, and experience through this joy and fulfillment.

Food, because we take it directly into our bodies on such a consistent basis, is one of the most powerful approaches to clearing the energy field to bring us closer to self-realization and optimum physical health.

THESE ARE THE FOODS WITH THE HIGHEST VIBRATION:

* Live or raw
* Fresh
* Organic or bio-dynamic
* Plant-based: vegetables, fruit, nuts, seeds, whole grains
* Grown and picked by people with high vibrations
* Prepared by people with high vibrations
* If you are eating animal products, know the source and be sure that the animals have been treated with compassion and respect.

Poor quality, processed, chemically-treated food negatively affects the human energy field. This becomes more and more obvious the more you refine your diet. You will become more aware of how unconscious food choices deflate your spirit, dull your mind, wreak havoc on your emotions, and deaden your physical body.

Through my health practice, I have come to realize that people often actually choose to stay in a state of half-aliveness and continue eating certain poor quality foods that keep them there. This is an unconscious choice, of course, but a very real and common phenomenon. One of the reasons for this is that as we make food and lifestyle choices that clear our energy fields, we begin to come to life, so to speak. Initially, during the transition phases, often we temporarily feel the psycho-spiritual pain that caused us to hide our Light in the first place, understandably bringing up much fear at times—a reason why it is so important to marry a consistent spiritual practice with our improved eating habits. It also explains why each person's dietary choices will be different depending on the emotional and spiritual shifts they are going through at the time, and why it is important to pace ourselves gently when making health changes. When emotional patterns come to our awareness—and they will when we embark on a path to self-realization—we must culture the ability to be a witness to these emotions as they come to the surface—non-judgmental, detached, and loving. The truth is that we are not our emotions, we are not our mind, we are not even our body. We have emotions, a mind and a body, but the truth of our being lies deeper in our pure Light. A regular spiritual practice helps us develop deep trust in the process. And we also know that there are many dedicated and gifted holistic health practitioners who can help us. We are never alone...

"Know your soul and you know all. It is in your soul where the origin of the world is. The Light of the soul is the illuminator of the universe. Let your love for and your loyalty to Truth, which is Existence – Consciousness – Bliss Absolute be first kindled within you at the bottom of your heart... Thirst for peace, and drink the pure nectar of real freedom in the life of Truth."
V.T. NEELAKANTAN IN MYSTICISM UNLOCKED (OF KRIYA BABAJI)

Your Spiritual Practice

Create an inviting place to sit, or an altar, using any of the following: a candle, some rocks, crystals or stones, feathers, pictures of spiritual teachers and/or people that you love, flowers, a prayer book, meaningful objects, hand-written intentions. Leave this place set up and spend some time there every day. At least 20 minutes twice a day is optimal. First thing in the morning and/or last thing at night. I like to sit for a while in the afternoon too.

Then do any of the following:

* STRETCH OR MOVE
  (*Suggestion*: Do a search for the Five Tibetan Rites of Rejuvenation on the internet. These are exercises that are quick, effective, and relatively easy to do. Or do a series of yoga stretches. The classic Sun Salutation series is balanced and beneficial.)

* BREATHE
  (simply be aware of your breath or use yoga pranayam techniques)

* SET FEELING-BASED INTENTIONS AND AFFIRMATIONS
  (Louise Hay's You Can Heal Your Life is an excellent resource for this)

* PRAY
  (use your own prayer or some other prayer that you know)

* SING OR CHANT

* MEDITATE

* BALANCE THE CHAKRAS

* FEEL

* LISTEN TO YOUR BODY

* READ INSPIRING LITERATURE

* ASK QUESTIONS AND RECEIVE ANSWERS

* LISTEN TO A GUIDED MEDITATION CD
  (you can order mine at www.carolinedupont.com)

"Honor your body, which is your representative in this universe. Its magnificence is no accident. It is the framework through which your works must come; through which the spirit and the spirit within the spirit speaks. The flesh and the spirit are two phases of your actuality in space and time. Who ignores one, falls apart in shambles. So it is written.

The marriage of soul and flesh is an ancient contract, to be honored.

Let no soul in flesh ignore its Earthly counterpart, or be unkind to its mate in time.

The mind cannot dance above the flesh, or on the flesh. It cannot deny the flesh or it turns into a demon demanding domination. Then the voice of the flesh cries out with yearning through all of its parts; the ancient contract undone. And both soul and flesh go begging, each alone and without partner.

Who feeds the body with love, neither starving nor stuffing it, feeds the soul. Who denies the body denies the soul. Who betrays it betrays the soul. The body is the body of the soul, the corporal image of knowledge. As men and women are married to each other, so is each self wedded to its body.

Those who do not love the body or trust it do not love or trust the soul. The multitudinous voices of the gods speak through the body parts. Even the golden molecules are not mute. Who muzzles the body or leashes it muzzles and leashes the soul. The private body is the dwelling place of the private guise of God. Do it honor. Let no man set himself up above the body, calling it soiled, for to him the splendor of the self is hidden. Let no one drive the body like a horse in captivity, to be ridden, or he will be trampled.

The body is the soul in Earth-garments. It is the face of the soul turned toward the seasons, the image of the soul reflected in Earth waters. The body is the soul turned outward. Soul and body are merged in the land of the seasons. Such is the ancient contract by which the Earth was formed.

The knowledge of the soul is written in the body. Body and soul are the inner and outer of the self. The spirit from which the soul springs forms both — soul and body. In Earth time, the soul and body learn together. The genes are the alphabets by which the soul speaks the body — which is the soul's utterance in flesh.

So let the soul freely speak itself in flesh.

The body is also eternal. The soul takes it out of space-time. The body is the soul's expression, and its expression is not finite. The spirit has many souls, and each has a body. The body is in and out of time, even as the soul is. Let the soul rush freely throughout the body, and breathe life into all of its parts. The first birth was a gift, freely given. Trust the spontaneity and the health of the body, which is the spontaneity and health of the soul. For each morning you spring anew, alive and fresh, out of chaos...."

THE EDUCATION OF OVERSOUL SEVEN BY JANE ROBERTS

Five Nutritional Guidelines
That Apply to Everyone

In the following sections I offer guidelines for the healthiest nutritional choices, for improved digestion, detoxification, weight loss, and healing. These are based on age-old philosophies, traditions that span generations, personal experience, intuition, and scientific research. Being a scientist, I can appreciate the importance of scientific research and rejoice when science proves what some of us have known intuitively and experientially all along. The more I experience though, the more I am willing to trust other ways that we acquire knowledge and truth because science often lags behind. Long ago, I decided that I wouldn't wait until people in white lab coats can prove what I can clearly experience for myself. I am learning to trust my intuition, my wisdom, my heart, and the subtle signals of my body. There are some things that need to be believed to be seen.

It is important that you, as a reader, also filter everything that you will read between these covers through your wisdom, your heart, and your intuition. Apply what feels right for you now and let the rest fall into place as it does. Health is a never-ending fascinating journey that will bring you rewards beyond currently accepted possibilities. At the core of each of our beings is the ability to be perfectly healthy in all realms, to be disease-free, and to reverse any disease that may be present at this time. Embrace these possibilities and watch all kinds of new information, people, workshops, and insights come into your life to support you along the way. Mostly, do it with dynamic ease—let the process be alive, effortless, and joyful. As the Tao says, do not use force to conquer the universe for this would only cause resistance. Force is followed by a loss of strength. So if you effort too much along your health path, you will become tired and disillusioned. From my own experience, most lasting shifts arise from inspiration. Inspiration: to be filled with spirit. A light goes on inside that simply says, "It is time." You are ready for this new shift, this new addition to your health practices. It could be juicing, or exercise, or eating less meat, or starting a meditation practice... and the universe supports you in as much as you take responsibility for yourself.

SO WITHOUT FURTHER ADO HERE IS SOME FOOD FOR THOUGHT:

"Eat, therefore, all your life at the table of our Earthly Mother, and you will never see want. And when you eat at her table, eat all things even as they are found on the table of the Earthly Mother." THE ESSENE GOSPEL OF PEACE, TRANSLATED BY EDMUND BORDEAUX SZÉKELY

1. Choose foods that are whole and in their natural state.

If you can incorporate this basic principle into your life, you will reap great benefits. What does "whole" mean? When you select a food, think about how it grows in nature; the closer you can get to that state the better. The Earth has been providing balanced wholesome foods since the beginning of time and will continue to do so if we allow Her to. Any time a food is processed, nutrients like vitamins, minerals, enzymes, and fiber are removed, creating a relative nutrient debt. If you want your billions of cells to function optimally, you need the nutrients that whole foods provide for you. Healthy cells create healthy organs, healthy systems, and a healthy body.

THIS MEANS THAT YOU WILL CHOOSE THE FOLLOWING FOODS MORE OFTEN:
* Raw, live foods
* Fresh vegetables
* Fresh fruit
* Nuts and seeds
* Whole grains
* Possibly, whole forms of animal products (dairy and eggs)

Some whole foods choices are not so obvious because we have been brainwashed by the media as to their healthfulness. For example, you should eat whole grains rather than white flour, bran, or wheat germ separately. If you are eating dairy, choose whole milk products, not skim. The fat is needed to absorb the minerals and to digest the protein. Eat legumes, not TVP (texturized vegetable protein found in many meat analogs). Remember, simply think about how it grows in nature and eat it as close to that state as possible. Nothing surpasses the wisdom of the Earth. Trust it.

2. Choose organic and bio-dynamic foods as often as possible.

ORGANIC FOODS:
* Have less or no chemicals. Organic farmers use no chemicals such as pesticides, herbicides, fungicides, or artificial fertilizers. However, because they don't farm in a bubble, there may be some small residues from other sources.
* Help to maintain the quality of the topsoil, the complex ecosystem including insects, soil-based organisms, humus, clay, and more that ultimately make up the living earth. Much of our topsoil is disappearing due to intensive industrial agriculture. How will we feed ourselves when the topsoil is gone?
* Have more minerals and other nutrients because the soil that they are grown in is replenished by the farmers on an ongoing basis. This has been supported by much research.
* Have more vibrant energy fields. This is supported by Kirlian photography which pictures objects as well as their energy field.
* Support family farms that are committed to maintaining the quality of the soil that our food is grown in and to minimizing their effect on the natural world. It takes only about 10 families eating organic to support one small-scale organic farm.

* Are the product of sustainable and morally responsible agriculture that ensures wholesome foods and a clean Earth for future generations.
* Increase agricultural diversity. Eating organic helps preserve thousands of agricultural varieties not accommodated by industrial agriculture.
* Taste better. Many top chefs know this and insist on organic ingredients.

Think about it—we simply cannot continue putting chemicals, that are designed to kill life, on our food and expect nature and our bodies to remain unaffected. These chemicals are bio-accumulating in our rivers, lakes, oceans, land, animal life, and our very own bodies, slowly poisoning the entire planet. There are many books written on this very important subject (Silent Spring, by Rachel Carson, was one of the first books to sound the alarm), but I know that every human being who simply uses his or her logic will clearly see the insanity of what we are doing to ourselves. In simple terms, these practices are not sustainable. We need to look in our hearts and reflect on what kind of legacy we want to leave for our children. There are many non-polluting options available today. In my heart, I know that the Earth can, and will, heal if we all do our part in making day-to-day choices as best we can to be part of the solution rather than adding to pollution.

Also, begin to consider adding more foods from heritage seeds, as well as selections from the wild. They have more nutritional value, brighter energy fields, and are hardy plants that don't require chemicals to fight off insects and weeds.

3. Choose food that is fresh, local, and seasonal.

* Food that is fresh maintains more of its nutrients and energy field.
* Local food is best suited for people who live in the environment where it was grown. Also, the transportation of imported foods creates tremendous amounts of pollution and greenhouse gases.
* Your dietary needs will vary according to the seasons. By eating locally and paying attention to your body's signals, you will find that the types of foods that bring you satisfaction will be different in the summer, fall, winter, and spring.

4. Choose a variety of foods, colours, flavours, textures, shapes, and directions of growth.

* VARIETY: alter your choices of grains, vegetables, fruit, nuts, and meats for interest, nutrient diversity, allergy prevention, and subtle qualities.
* COLOURS: daily, choose foods from the whole spectrum of colours for energetic qualities, nutrient diversity, and visual appeal.
* FLAVOURS: enjoy all of the six flavours—sweet, sour, salty, bitter, astringent, pungent. Most single foods consist of various flavours, one being predominant. In Ayurvedic philosophy, flavours bring psycho-spiritual qualities with them, and in order to be balanced physically and spiritually we should include all of them in our diets on a daily basis, preferably at one meal. When creating your own

recipes, think about how you can include all of the flavours—you will notice a greater satisfaction from consuming dishes this way. At the beginning of some of my recipes, I indicate which foods contribute the various flavours.

Here are some examples of how foods fit into flavour categories:

- *Sweet foods include:* most grains like rice and wheat, sweet fruit, carrots, beets, many nuts, honey, milk, cream, butter. Meats and fish are also considered sweet.
- *Sour foods include:* lemons, tomatoes, grapes, plums, and other sour fruit, cheese, yogourt, and vinegar.
- *Salty foods* have a salty flavour, for example, seaweed, celery, some leafy greens, or any food with added salt.
- *Bitter foods include:* green leafy vegetables, endive, chicory, romaine lettuce, parsley, coriander, coffee.
- *Pungent foods include:* cayenne, chili peppers, onions, garlic, leeks, radishes, ginger, and spicy foods in general.
- *Astringent (dry sensation in the mouth) foods include:* beans, lentils, apples, pears, cabbage, broccoli, cauliflower, potatoes, some nuts.

* TEXTURES: soft, crunchy, chewy, watery, smooth, granular—select a variety.

* SHAPE: be creative when preparing and cutting foods.

* DIRECTION OF GROWTH: regularly choose vegetables that grow upwards (leafy greens), downwards (carrots, yams), sideways (squash), hanging (beans, peas).

5. Conscious eating: Awareness leads to insight; insight leads to clarity; clarity leads to freedom...

The ideal way to individualize a diet that will give you optimum health, vitality, and longevity is to become more conscious of how your food choices affect all aspects of your life. Your body will give you all kinds of signals and clues as to the best nutritional choices—all you have to do, as the body's owner and best expert, is to listen as attentively as possible. The only tricky part is the timing of the reaction to the particular food. Sometimes just the thought of a food will give you subtle body reactions, or you will feel effects as soon as you put it on your tongue, or 30 minutes after you eat it, or up to 3 or 4 days after you eat it (particularly with arthritis). The more you pay attention and practice awareness, the more attuned you will be to the effects of foods on your physical body and your energy field. Recently I was stirring a chocolate fondue at my parents' place and an unpleasant pressure began in my head similar to when I had eaten chocolate in the past. Another time, after I had eaten only raw foods for several days, I ate a cooked cob of corn (probably genetically engineered) and immediately felt the dulling of my mind. At times when I go shopping at the local health food store, I am strongly drawn to certain foods even if I have never eaten them before.

* THE QUALITY OF YOUR SLEEP: Note times awakened, depth of sleep, dreams, thoughts, ease in falling asleep.
* HOW YOU FEEL FIRST THING IN THE MORNING: Note how rested you feel, how your body feels, stiff joints, stuffed or runny nose, energy level, enthusiasm for the new day, predominant emotions, how your face looked (check eyes, skin, tongue).
* HOW YOU FEEL THE REST OF THE DAY:
  Physically: Note general energy level, specific areas of discomfort, cold hands/feet, allergies.
  Mentally: Note mental alertness, awareness, quality of thought patterns, speed of thoughts, ability to make decisions, clarity.
  Emotionally: Note ability to feel emotions, as well as specific emotions, emotions that got out of control, quality of relationships.
  Spiritually: Note connection with your higher God-self, with Earth, with your own core energy, degree of centeredness, awareness of your purpose and your essence, connection to others and to the Whole.
* BOWEL MOVEMENTS: Note time, frequency, quality (feces too hard or too soft), ease of elimination.
* HOW YOU FEEL RELATIVE TO EACH MEAL:
  Note level of hunger before eating, enjoyment of eating, any emotions, thought patterns, energy level before and after eating (it should not drop), level of satiety, digestive system discomfort (gas, bloating, indigestion), mental alertness, change in heart rate (more than 20 beats per minute increase 30 minutes after a meal may signal an allergy), fatigue.

Note any ideas, thoughts, and intuitions that you may have gained by eating consciously, as well as modifications you will want to try... This is an important step. What have you learned?

"Do not fight against circumstances.
Your face ought to shine.
Your spirit ought to be tranquil.
Your eye ought to be clear.
Your nerves ought to be steady.
With these, press through the tasks of your
most common day.
Live as finely and beautifully in private
as in the open glare of the world's noon.
Train yourself to work under the Divine eye
and stand the Divine inspection.
Let the life begin to stir from the innermost depths
and richly yield its true measure of joyfulness."

WEEKLY MESSAGE FROM BABJI'S KRIYA YOGA #174

The New Food Groups

The following guidelines for daily food selection are general and could be adjusted in the case of disease or food sensitivities, but for most people this is an excellent foundation for superior health. The number of servings will vary according to size and activity level. Eat to satisfy your hunger.

Fruit and vegetables – 70 to 80% of food intake

* Fresh fruit: 2 or more servings per day (increase on a living foods diet – can vary but 10 or more servings per day is not rare among living food advocates). Eat fruit alone or with juicy vegetables like lettuce or celery.
* Include 3 or more servings of raw vegetables every day, as is, or in a salad.
* Include a total of at least 4 servings of vegetables every day: at least 1 serving of green vegetables and 1 serving of orange vegetables every day.
* Include a variety of fresh fruit, preferably organic.
* Focus on fruit in season, but if you're tending towards a raw diet you will be including tropical and semi-tropical fruit.
* Vegetables should be fresh (not canned or frozen) and eaten raw or cooked.
* Include sea vegetables and sprouts more often.

Whole grains

* 2 to 5 servings every day
* Focus on gluten-free whole grains (not flour products): brown rice, quinoa, millet, buckwheat.
* Choose alternatives to wheat more often: kamut, spelt, oats, etc.
* Choose sprouted grain products more often.
* For living food diets, this category can be omitted altogether or you could make dehydrated spouted grain crackers and breads, or raw porridges.

Proteins

* at least 2 servings per day
* Legumes: at least 1 serving every day
* Dairy (optional) – if no sensitivities: 1 serving every 2 days
* Eggs (optional): 1 or 2 per week
* For living foods diets, this category could be omitted but you would have to compensate with more vegetables and fruit.

Fats and oils

* Nuts and seeds: 1 serving per day
* Nut and seed butters (optional): maximum 1 Tbs. per day
* Cold-pressed oils: 1 Tbs. per day used in cooking or salads
* Fatty fruit (avocado, olives): 1 serving per day

"Breathe long and deep at all your meals,
that the angel of air may bless your repasts.
And chew well your food with your teeth,
that it become water,
and that the angel of water turn it into blood in your body.
And eat slowly, as it were a prayer you make to the Lord.
... And enter only into the Lord's sanctuary
when you feel in yourselves the call of his angels,
for all that you eat in sorrow, or in anger, or without desire,
becomes a poison in your body...
And never sit at the table of God
before he calls you by the angel of appetite."

THE ESSENE GOSPEL OF PEACE

Digestion: Differentiating Diet and Nutrition

Diet is what you put into your mouth and nutrition is what actually gets into the billions of cells in your body. The limiting and enabling factor is digestion. Most people actually digest very little of what they eat because their digestive system is under-functioning due to years of eating poor quality foods and stress. What doesn't get digested ferments in the intestines, introduces toxins into the bloodstream, feeds yeasts and parasites, and creates layers of buildup on the walls of the intestines (called mucoid plaque), further decreasing absorption. What follows are some guidelines to enable the building of digestive fire so that the food you take in is thoroughly absorbed. There is little point in spending time and money on selecting high quality food if you do not also consider how to improve its absorption.

Eat in a calm, relaxed state

All digestive system functions, from secretion of saliva and pancreatic juice to absorption through intestinal walls, to the work of the liver and the kidneys, are governed by the parasympathetic nervous system. The other branch of the nervous system is the sympathetic nervous system, which governs the stress response (also known as fight or flight). When the sympathetic nervous system is on, the parasympathetic shuts off. In other words, you cannot be stressed and digest well at the same time! For the same reason, you should avoid eating when you are emotionally upset. Most of us live much of our lives in an elevated sympathetic state and so we need to develop a relaxation practice, like meditation, to re-learn how to easily shift back into parasympathetic mode and eventually live more of our days in this relaxed state. It is not enough to simply tell ourselves to relax when we eat. Like a puppy who needs to be trained, our bodies need a daily spiritual practice so that we can access these relaxed states easily when we are in stress mode. Of course, this same spiritual practice will give us an abundance of other gifts as well.

Chew thoroughly

Chewing your food to a paste breaks it into very small particles, making it more accessible by food enzymes. It also stimulates the secretion of saliva and carbohydrate digesting enzymes in the mouth.

Eat only when hungry

This is an obvious one—rather than eating by the clock we need to listen to our hunger signals. This may even mean sometimes skipping a meal or eating less than usual. When hunger is felt in the back of the throat, our stomachs feel relaxed and we salivate easily at the thought or sight of food—we are hungry. Sometimes thirst masquerades as hunger, so drink plenty of water.

Avoid overeating

Eat slowly and stop eating before you are full. Excessive food places strain on the digestive system and will not be fully broken down and absorbed. Overeating is one of the greatest physical and spiritual energy robbers. Many studies of groups of people who have the greatest longevity find that they typically eat 50% fewer calories than North Americans. When rats are fed 40% less food they live 40% longer. There are studies being conducted at various universities that are showing a decrease in biological age when people adopt a frugal eating style. It is important to eat only the best quality food when reducing calories.

Avoid drinking large quantities of liquid, especially cold, when eating

The best time to drink fluids is between meals. Large quantities of fluid dilute the digestive enzymes that your body secretes, and cold liquids decrease the temperature of the parietal cells of the stomach which slows down their metabolism. Small sips of fresh juice or room temperature water are fine.

Keep meals simple, not mixing too many different foods together

The fewer types of food, the less complicated it is for the digestive system. Mono meals (one type of food) are great sometimes too. Try eating simpler meals and see for yourself how much better you feel. You don't have to get all of your required nutrients at one meal. As long as over the course of the week and the year you eat a wide variety of foods, you'll get all that you need.

Have at least some raw, uncooked food with every meal

Cooked foods (above 118F) require the input of large amounts of digestive enzymes along the entire length of the digestive system, whereas raw foods, particularly fruit, are already pre-digested when eaten ripe.

Food combine, especially if digestion is weak

There are many principles of food combining from the Natural Hygiene approach popularized by Harvey and Marilyn Diamond in their book Fit For Life. The two main guidelines are: eat fruit alone because it digests so much more quickly than any other food, and avoid mixing concentrated proteins and starches at a meal. A concentrated protein is meat or dairy, and a concentrated starch is a grain or potato. So you would avoid having fish and potatoes, or a chicken sandwich, or spaghetti and meatballs. The digestive requirements of these two groups of foods are vastly different and compete with each other, hindering complete digestion and taxing our organs. So, one day you could have a big salad with feta cheese or chick peas for dinner, and the next day you could have brown rice with vegetables. Vegetables, in general, combine well with any foods. There are many good books and guides for food combining. Check out the works of Herbert Shelton, T.C. Fry, or Arnold Ehret. Vegetarians don't have to worry too much about food combining, particularly if they are not eating dairy or eggs (concentrated proteins). However, some people will want to avoid mixing legumes (considered by some to be a concentrated protein – and it's also high starch) with grains. On the other hand, many cultures have been eating grains and legumes together for a long time because they intuitively knew that the proteins contained in these two groups of foods complement each other and create a more complete protein. So the Central and South Americans eat corn and pinto beans, the East Indians eat rice and dahl (a soupy lentil or mung bean mixture), some Africans eat millet and chick peas, etc. As always, the best is to try it out for yourself and see how you feel.

Fast at least 14 hours per day

This break from eating gives your digestive system a rest, gives you time to build digestive fire, and allows for more thorough detoxification. Prolonged fasting, when you are ready, is also very helpful for deeper detoxification.

Practice conscious eating, connecting to your food with all of your senses and a grateful attitude

Sit down. Avoid distractions like the phone, television, computer or loud music. Appreciate the smell, the look, the colours, the feel, the texture, the taste, and other aspects of the food you are eating. In this way, food consumption becomes a richer, fuller experience. It's more than simply filling our stomachs. A grateful approach opens the heart and the entire being to receiving, and creates an attitude where it's possible to consistently make health-supporting choices, to feel satisfied with less, and to truly enjoy eating—letting go of battles that we may have been struggling with for years.

Bless your food

"The words and gestures of the blessing wrap the food in emanations and fluids which prepare it to vibrate in harmony with you who are going to eat it, and an adaptation happens in your subtle bodies which enables you to receive and benefit from all the properties contained in the food." OMRAAM MIKHAËL AÏVANHOV IN THE YOGA OF NUTRITION

Use candles, special dishes, flowers, table settings, and more to create beauty around meal time

Why wait for guests to take out special dishes? Beauty helps us slow down and appreciate our meals, creates a pleasant atmosphere around the dinner table, opens the heart and the energy field to receiving, and leads to effortlessly making health-supporting choices.

Supplementing a Whole-foods Diet

The key to radiant health is to enjoy the best quality food that you can find. Please focus on establishing this practice and know that while supplements have limited intelligence, they fall short of the wisdom of whole natural foods. Often, because many supplements are made up of isolated nutrients (like vitamins or minerals), they can cause imbalances within the body, which is designed to take in a wide variety of nutrients found in perfect balance in nature's foods. For example, if you are taking a calcium-magnesium supplement to protect from osteoporosis there is a mechanism in the body governed by the parathyroid gland that will shut down the absorption of these minerals from food as the blood levels get high from the unnatural amounts in the supplement. Also, we need many other nutrients besides calcium and magnesium to build strong bones, like boron, silica, sulfur and zinc, and vitamins A, D and E, as well as protein and essential amino acids. All of these can be obtained in absorbable and balanced forms from whole organic foods. Another faulty thought pattern is that more of any nutrient is necessarily better. Yet, this is never the case. The body only needs what it needs. The rest must be excreted by the organs of elimination, overloading them with another avoidable task.

THE ONLY SUPPLEMENTS THAT I RECOMMEND ARE FRESH PRESSED JUICES AND SUPERFOOD POWDERS AND LIQUIDS:

Fresh pressed juices

Fresh pressed juices are, in my opinion, the ultimate supplement to any diet. At this stage in our collective health journey, juices are the universal supplement. Why?

* Most of us have nutrient deficiencies, especially in the mineral category.
* Most of us have poor digestion.
* Many supplements (vitamin/mineral pills) are not easily digested and absorbed, and may even cause nutrient imbalances by competing with other nutrients.
* Fresh pressed juices are made up of whole foods in perfect nutritional balance, and will be absorbed from the stomach and upper intestine minutes after ingestion. You can be sure that the nutrients from the carrot, kale, celery, lemon, and apple contained in your late-afternoon juice will get to your cells and contribute to the rebuilding of your system and to detoxification. Plus, fresh juice contains living enzymes which assist in virtually every physiological function of the body.
* Most people will feel the energizing effects of juice soon after starting this practice; and within a week of juicing regularly, generally energy levels noticeably increase.

People often ask what kind of juicer is best. The most important factor for many people is how much they are willing to spend. Many products can be purchased at your local department store for approximately $100. The plus is the price. The minus is the fact that some machines will heat your produce through friction, destroying nutrients. Some do not extract as much juice as possible and the pulp is still quite moist (you could feed it through again). Many are hard to clean and that will discourage you from making fresh juice. If you are juicing a lot, you may burn out the motor in a short time.

My first juicer was a Champion and it served me well for 12 years. This is a high quality, sturdy juicer/grinder which will do a great job juicing anything except the grasses. I found that it did heat the produce sometimes, especially when I was doing a lot of greens. The price is relatively reasonable considering the quality. You can get a Champion for $350 to $400 (Canadian funds). The motor on these machines will last a lifetime and you can order new parts (occasionally blades need to be replaced).

Recently I bought a twin-gear Green Power Juicer for $700. It does an excellent job on greens and hard vegetables like carrots, a good job on grasses, and an average job on fruit. It works well for me because I primarily juice greens and vegetables; it doesn't heat the produce at all because of its slow rotation speed; and I can still use it for grinding patés and ice creams. There are other excellent quality twin-gear juicers on the market.

Green Powders

Green powders are probably the most popular way of supplementing a whole foods diet. Unless you're juicing and consistently using organic produce, I feel that they are necessary at this stage. These products are primarily made from freeze-dried super-foods (i.e., foods that are known to contain high concentrations of various nutrients, for example, barley or wheat grass, spirulina, chlorella, and blue-green algae). Many manufacturers market formulas that contain a variety of ingredients (often as many as 70 different ingredients). There are many products available, some excellent, some not as high quality.

THINGS TO CONSIDER WHEN CHOOSING A GREEN POWDER:
* Single ingredient powders (or tablets and capsules) are often the best way to ensure high concentrations of a product, and are usually more cost-effective. Look for spirulina, chlorella, wheat-grass powder, barley-grass powder, and blue-green algae among others. There are also frozen liquid forms of most of these available.
* Multi-ingredient powders are proprietary formulas which may contain algae, grass powders, probiotics, herbs, mushrooms, vegetable powders, and fillers.
* Beware of inexpensive fillers like lecithin, pectin, and rice bran (you will be fooled into thinking that you are getting more product than you think).
* I have some reservations about the addition of herbs to green powders. First, we don't all have the same needs when it comes to herbal supplementation. These needs depend on constitution and current health status. Second, herbs are meant to be taken over short periods and then stopped. The body adapts and the herb ceases having its initial effect.

* Some powders add so-called natural flavourings. I personally find these obnoxious and many people notice that they get sick of these products quickly.
* If you react to a multi-ingredient powder, it is very hard to determine the exact source of the sensitivity. Try a single ingredient powder.
* In this case, it's true that the more expensive powders are usually the best quality.
* When purchasing supplements, ask a nutritionist for advice on the best brands and make sure that they are coming from natural sources. Many good products are available, but they can be expensive. I would much rather see someone spend an extra $100 per month on better quality foods than on supplements.

Anti-nutrients

As important as it is to choose natural, alive, and high quality foods, and to ensure proper digestion, you also want to consider certain practices that destroy precious nutrients (vitamins, essential fatty acids, minerals, and enzymes) once they are in our bodies, or cause us to excrete excessive quantities of these nutrients, or prevent us from absorbing them.

The following is a list of anti-nutrients. There aren't too many surprises – most of them are known to be counter to health by most of the population. Try to reduce or eliminate them as much as possible.

* physical, mental, emotional, and spiritual stress
* lack of exercise
* lack of sleep
* refined foods like white sugar and white flour
* caffeine (coffee and black tea)
* excess animal protein
* smoking
* alcohol
* prescription and recreational drugs
* some supplements
* antibiotics
* birth control pills
* soft drinks
* overeating
* chemicals: tap water, household cleaners, cosmetics, etc.

"The body is the sacred sanctuary of the soul. Care for it like you would a flower garden. Only when you honor, love and cherish your body can your spirit soar." ILANA RUBENFELD

Detoxification

" ... And when all sins and uncleanness are gone from your body, your blood shall become as pure as our Earthly Mother's blood and as the river's foam sporting in the sunlight. And your breath shall become as pure as the breath of odorous flowers; your flesh as pure as the flesh of fruits reddening upon the leaves of trees; the light of your eye as clear and bright as the brightness of the sun shining upon the blue sky." ESSENE GOSPEL OF PEACE (EGP), BOOK 1

Signs and symptoms of toxicity

* aches and pains (arthritis, gout, stiff muscles and joints, low back pains, fibromyalgia)
* poor skin quality (acne, boils, eczema, psoriasis, dryness)
* coated tongue
* circles/bags under the eyes
* headaches (sinus, tension, migraine)
* allergies (sinus inflammation, congestion, itchy eyes and skin)
* emotional instability (anxiety, depression, mood swings)
* negative mind patterns (inability to concentrate, overactive mind, negative thoughts, closed-mindedness)
* fatigue (inability to fall asleep, to sleep soundly, to feel rested)
* poor digestion (bloating, acid reflux, gas, pain, nausea)
* diseases of the digestive system (Crohn's, colitis, diverticulitis, irritable bowel, gallstones)
* female cycle disturbances (painful periods, PMS, menopausal symptoms, irregular periods, fibroids, cysts)
* hypertension
* diabetes (childhood and adult onset)
* respiratory disturbances (coughing, wheezing, asthma, bronchitis, emphysema)
* constipation
* overweight
* cardiovascular disease (heart attacks, strokes, claudication)
* mental disease (Parkinson's, Alzheimer's, senility)
* infections (bacteria, viruses, fungus, parasites)
* addictions (drugs, coffee, alcohol)
* etc.

On the positive side

This is how you will feel when your body is purified (to greater degrees as you go through the process):

* Physical energy and vitality
* Balanced bodily rhythms: digestion, elimination, sleep, female cycle
* Strong disease immunity
* Mental and emotional clarity
* Enhanced intuition and knowing
* More consistent ability to connect to spirit
* Underlying level of peace

Exogenous and endogenous toxins

Know where the toxins are coming from and avoid them.
EXOGENOUS: enter through mouth (food, water), skin (water, creams), and lungs (air). Includes poor quality food (refined and processed – especially fats and oils, sugar, and white flour), pesticides, food additives, preservatives, tap water, household cleaners, outgases from construction and home decorating, industrial pollution, cosmetics, amalgam fillings, plastics, air fresheners, perfumes, microwave ovens, teflon coated cookware, and radiation. Also noise pollution and information overload (television, newspapers, radio, books).
ENDOGENOUS: by-products of digestion, putrefying food residues, cellular wastes, fungal (candida) and parasite waste products, and acidity (acid-forming foods, negative thoughts and emotions).

The 5 physiological processes of nourishment

1. INGESTION: the taking in of food.
2. DIGESTION: the breaking down of food within the digestive tract, with the help of digestive fluids and enzymes.
3. ABSORPTION: the absorption of macro and micro nutrients into the blood and the cells.
4. ASSIMILATION: the utilization of the nutrients by the cells for building, repair and maintenance.
5. DETOXIFICATION AND EGESTION: the excretion of by-products of digestion and metabolism through the various routes of elimination.

THE LESS ENERGY WE SPEND ON INGESTION, DIGESTION, ABSORPTION, AND ASSIMILATION, THE MORE ENERGY WE HAVE AVAILABLE FOR DETOXIFICATION.

Therefore, any detoxification regime encourages the increased removal of toxins by emphasizing one or more of the following:

* Ingestion of highest quality foods possible
* Ingestion of foods that are easy to digest, focusing on fruit and vegetables (raw and steamed) with some gluten-free grains, legumes and nuts and seeds
* Following guidelines for proper digestion
* Practicing techniques that encourage removal of toxins from the various routes
  More to come...

Signs and symptoms of detoxification (healing crisis)

When you think you're getting worse, know that there are various symptoms that are possible as the body heals and eliminates toxins. Here are some of them:

* Headaches
* Body aches and pains
* Diarrhea
* Skin eruptions
* Coated tongue
* Dark urine
* Body odour
* Dizziness
* Weakness
* Fever
* Return of past symptoms

Of course, when in doubt, speak to your natural health practitioner.

Hering's law of cure

Your body is ever so wise—when cared for, it will heal in its own time and its own way. However, generally the body heals:

* From the inside out. For example, a digestive issue will balance before a skin condition does.
* From the top down. For example, a sinus issue will heal before arthritis in the knee.
* From most recent to most distant symptoms. For example, the gallstones that developed three years ago will pass before the colitis that started 15 years ago heals.
* From the more important organs to the less important ones. For example, the liver will heal before the spleen.

Levels of Dietary Detoxification

In general, choose less congesting and potentially toxic foods.

MOST CONGESTING:

drugs, allergenic foods, organ meats, hydrogenated fats, fried foods, refined flours, meats, baked goods, sugar, milk, eggs.

MODERATELY CONGESTING:

nuts, seeds, legumes, grains, starchy vegetables

LEAST CONGESTING:

fruit, vegetables, greens, sprouts, herbs, water

A. General detoxification diet/maintenance diet – Level 1

This diet will be detoxifying for most people who are currently eating an average North American diet. It emphasizes high quality whole foods.

* Organic
* Fresh
* Local and seasonal
* Delicious and satisfying
* Conscious choices
* Balanced:
   Variety of foods: vegetables, fruit, nuts and seeds, sprouts, whole grains, legumes, possibly animal products
   Variety of colours: red, orange, yellow, green, purple/blue, white
   Variety of flavours: sweet, sour, salty, bitter, astringent, pungent
   Variety of textures and shapes

FOOD SELECTION

Beverages: Pure water, fresh pressed vegetable and fruit juices, herbal teas, nut milks, rice milk, natural coffee substitutes.

Dairy (if no sensitivities): Organic, raw, not homogenized when possible, yogourt, kefir, cheeses, full fat.

Fruit: Fresh fruit and berries, focusing on seasonal, preferably tree-ripened, choose fruit with seeds when possible.

Grains, cereals, flour products: Emphasize gluten-free whole grains: brown rice, quinoa, millet, buckwheat, amaranth. For glutenous grains focus on sprouted products. Whole wheat, kamut, spelt. Also oats, rye and barley can be eaten in whole form. Choose sourdough and sprouted breads. Limit baked goods regardless of the grain.

Legumes: All kinds, dried are preferred over canned. Chick peas, pinto beans, kidney beans, lentils, split peas, etc. Use in soups and dips. Limited tofu and tempeh if no sensitivities to soy.

Nuts and seeds: Most raw or soaked nuts and seeds, except peanuts (insist on organic if you are buying any peanut products).

Oils and fats: Cold pressed oils – olive, hemp, flaxseed, sesame, sunflower, coconut. For frying – clarified butter (ghee), coconut oil. Olive oil and sesame oil, being mono-unsaturated are fine for light frying. Avoid corn oil, canola oil, processed oils (sunflower, safflower, soyabean oil), margarine.

Spices and condiments: Sea salt, pepper, herbs, garlic, ginger, onions. Natural catsup, mustard, and mayonnaise occasionally. Tamari (wheat-free is preferable), Bragg's Liquid Seasoning.

Sweeteners: Limited amounts of maple syrup, honey, agave syrup, molasses, granulated sugar cane juice (sucanat), barley malt, rice syrup.

Vegetables: All in unlimited amounts, raw, in salads, lightly steamed, soups. Avoid corn if it is a sensitivity.

B. General detoxification diet – Level 2

This diet is a step beyond the Level 1 diet because it eliminates all animal products and glutenous grains. It can be followed for a limited period of time to enhance detoxification, or can be used as a base point for an elimination diet. It can also be followed indefinitely with excellent health benefits, as long as care is taken to take mostly organic foods with attention to good protein sources (legumes, grains, greens, sprouts, nuts, and seeds) and B12 (supplementation or fermented foods).

If using this diet as a starting point for an elimination diet, follow it for 1 week or until symptoms subside. Then add one new food every 2 to 4 days. If symptoms re-occur with any particular food, eliminate it for 4 to 6 months and then try again, choosing the highest quality version that you can find.

* Eat only fresh fruit and vegetables, either raw or steamed. Unlimited amounts.
* Eat the following grains on a rotating basis: brown rice, quinoa, millet, buckwheat (kasha).
* Eat raw (and/or soaked) nuts and seeds in moderation. Make nut milks with these. (No peanuts.)
* Completely avoid animal products such as meat, poultry, dairy, fish, and eggs.

* Completely avoid all flour products and glutenous grains (includes wheat, spelt, kamut, oats, rye).
* Possibly use sprouted grain breads (self-test): Ezekiel 4:9 products, Nature's Path Manna Bread, Stickling's Total Value bread – these do contain some gluten (spelt, kamut, wheat) but the sprouting process breaks it down making it easier to digest.
* Completely avoid coffee, caffeinated teas, alcohol, tobacco, teas with natural flavours and colourings.
* Do not use any vitamin or mineral supplements.
* Drink fresh juice daily.

C. Living foods diet

This diet can be, and has been, followed for a limited period of time with excellent detoxification effects, or, with proper research and awareness, can be followed indefinitely.

"Therefore, eat not anything which fire, or frost, or water has destroyed. For burned, frozen and rotted foods will burn, freeze and rot your body also." EGP 1

GENERALLY
Eat raw fruit and vegetables, fresh pressed juices, nuts and seeds, sprouts, possibly sprouted grains, possibly raw dairy.

SPECIFICALLY
Wait until you are hungry in the morning. Then…
Breakfast and/or lunch: fruit, fruit salad, fresh fruit juice, fruit smoothies, green smoothies, soaked nuts and seeds, raw porridge
Lunch and dinner: more fruit, salads, nori rolls, pâtés, fresh juices, raw soups, sprouted nuts, seeds, sprouted grains, dehydrated foods, various vegetable dishes, raw crackers, avocados
Snacks: fruit, raw cookies and rolls, crackers, raw vegetables, dips, soaked nuts and seeds, sprouts, fresh juices or smoothies, sprouted bread

D. Blended foods, smoothies, and soups

* Incorporate into detoxification or living foods diets, or do 1 or more days on blended foods only.
* Excellent introduction to fasting for people with hypoglycemia, bowel disorders, constipation.
* Make various fruit-based smoothie or vegetable-based blended soup concoctions using soaked nuts and seeds, fruit juices, whole fruit or berries, nut milks, sprouts, vegetables and vegetable juices, avocados, and green powders.
* You will find recipes in this book (as well as most raw and living food recipe books).

E. Juice fast and/or Master Cleanse

Drink 2 to 5 fresh green juices per day or the Master Cleanse formula for 1 or more days.

BASIC GREEN JUICE (SEE IDEAS IN THE RECIPE SECTION):
50% greens: cucumber, celery, sunflower sprouts, buckwheat sprouts, kale, dandelion, spinach, parsley, cabbage, lettuce, wheatgrass
25% other vegetables: carrots, beets, tomatoes, parsley root, burdock root
25% fruit: apple, lemon, orange, pear, pineapple
Can also add ginger, garlic, herbs.

MASTER CLEANSE FORMULA:
2 Tbs. lemon juice
pinch cayenne pepper
1 to 2 Tbs. maple syrup
8 ounces purified water

MODIFIED MASTER CLEANSE:
2 Tbs. lemon juice
1 Tbs. raw honey
1 tsp. fresh grated ginger
8 ounces purified water

F. Water fast

"Go by yourself and fast alone, and show your fasting to no man. The living God shall see it and great shall be your reward... Fast and pray fervently, seeking the power of the living God for your healing." EGP 1

THE MOST POTENTIALLY DETOXIFYING CLEANSE, BUT ALSO MAY HAVE THE MOST ACUTE HEALING CRISIS – THESE USUALLY SUBSIDE WITHIN 3 DAYS.

* Make sure that you have established a consistently healthy diet for at least 6 months first.
* It is wise to do blended cleanses and juice fasts first.
* Also work into a water fast in the following manner:
  Normal diet (ideally similar to the detoxification diet mentioned above).
  One day raw fruit and vegetables as well as juices.
  Start the water fast.
* Work out of the fast in the following way – MOST IMPORTANT
  Break the fast with a fairly fibrous fruit, like apples, pears, melons, grapes, peaches, pineapple, mangos.
* For the first part of breaking the fast, take only raw fruit and raw and steamed vegetables. Do this for half the duration of the fast. For example, if the water fast lasted 7 days, then eat only fruit and vegetables for 3 or 4 days.
* It can be helpful to do enemas during a juice or water fast. See the section on specifics for the colon below.

How long should you fast for?

There are many possible answers. First of all, consult an experienced nutritionist or health practitioner. By "experienced", I mean someone who has studied fasting and has done some fasting themselves. Some say that you could go to a fasting centre and immediately go into a supervised 1 to 3 week water fast. I did my first 3-day water fast when I developed pneumonia near the beginning of my transition to a holistic diet. At the time I was 6 weeks pregnant. Amazingly, by the end of the 3 days the pneumonia cleared, as did the morning sickness I had been experiencing. After that I mainly did juice fasts throughout the year for periods of time varying from 1 day to 5 days. My second water fast was done about 13 years after my first one, for 8 days, between Christmas and New Years Day. In many ways, I found water fasting easier than any other type of cleanse that I have done. Although I did feel weak, and had various symptoms arise, I didn't feel hungry after the first day, and I felt very clear mentally and emotionally. By the 7th day, I felt that I would like to go on longer—my body seemed to want to continue. Because I was going back to work and my teenagers had returned home, I needed to get back to my regular schedule and could no longer move at the slower pace that I had adopted during my fast. It's best to rest completely when water fasting. That means no work, minimal exercise, and as much sleep as needed—therefore you need to plan a fast well in advance so that you can completely clear your schedule.

"... fasting in a larger context, means to abstain from that which is toxic to the mind, body, and soul. A way to understand this is that fasting is the elimination of physical, emotional, and mental toxins from our organism, rather than simply cutting down on or stopping food intake. Fasting for spiritual purposes usually involves some degree of removal of oneself from worldly responsibilities. It can mean complete silence and social isolation during the fast which can be a great revival to those of us who have been putting our energy outward."

SPIRITUAL NUTRITION AND THE RAINBOW DIET BY GABRIEL COUSENS

When to Cleanse/Fast

The best time to fast is when your health is suffering, and/or when you feel called to. Your body will begin to tell you in various ways that it needs to fast or cleanse.

HERE ARE SOME OF THE SIGNALS TO LOOK FOR:

* Food doesn't taste very good to you.
* Nothing is appetizing.
* Your digestion is poor.
* You are feeling tired.
* You are feeling like you are getting sick.
* You simply wake up one morning knowing that you need to cleanse.

General guidelines

ONCE PER WEEK:
Choose one day to fast or simply to eliminate the most congesting foods in your regular diet. For example, if you regularly eat dairy and wheat, eliminate those one day a week.

"On the seventh day eat not any earthly food, but live only on the words of God, and be all the day with the angels of the Lord in the kingdom of the Heavenly Father." EGP 1

ONCE PER SEASON:
3 days at the change of each season

ONCE PER YEAR:
7 or more days

Fasting setting

* No television, radio, newspapers
* Turn off phone
* Be in silence for at least part of the fast
* Take time off work
* Rest as much as you need to
* Spend plenty of time outdoors in sunshine and fresh air
* Increase your time spent in spiritual practice: meditation, prayer, breathwork, self-healing, body awareness exercises
* Movement: none or very light

Routes of Elimination-Detoxification Systems

Colon and small intestine

BEFORE PROCEEDING with any kind of liquid fast make sure that you are having at least 2 bowel movements per day. The colon and small intestine are the first organs to cleanse before proceeding to liquid fasts.

* Eat a high fibre, whole foods diet, plenty of high water content foods (fruit and vegetables).
* Be aware of foods that constipate you.
* Certain herbs can help to increase regularity and cleanse the intestines. You can find these and products containing them at your local health food store.
  Laxative herbs: cascara sagrada, dandelion, rhubarb root, barberry bark
  Demulcent herbs (remove mucus coating and replace with a lighter, cleaner mucilaginous coating): marshmallow root, flax seed, fenugreek seed, psyllium seed, licorice root.
* Here are some foods that lubricate the intestines: spinach, banana, sesame seed/oil, honey, pear, prune, peach, apple, apricot, walnut, pine nut, almond, alfalfa sprouts, soy products, carrot, cauliflower, beet, okra, whole fresh milk, seaweed.
* Here are some foods that promote bowel movement: cabbage, papaya, peas, black sesame seed, coconut, sweet potato, asparagus, fig, whole grains.
* Eat foods that enhance the good bacteria in your intestines: miso, sauerkraut, yogourt, kefir, chlorophyll-rich foods (wheat grass products, dark greens, micro-algae, sunflower, buckwheat, and other sprouts).
* Take probiotics, especially if you have recently taken antibiotics.
* Whenever doing a juice or water fast it can be helpful to do an enema once or twice per day.

"So I tell you truly, suffer the angel of water to baptize you also within ... Seek therefore, a large trailing gourd, having a stalk the length of a man; take out its inwards and fill it with water from the river which the sun has warmed. Hang it upon the branch of a tree, and kneel upon the ground before the angel of water, and suffer the end of the stalk of the trailing gourd to enter your hinder parts, that the water may flow through all your bowels." EGP 1

* It can be helpful to use Robert Gray's formula and program for removing mucoid matter from the intestinal tract before proceeding to juice and water fasts. His book is called the Colon Heath Handbook and the formula that he created has been marketed by Innovite under the brand name Holistic Horizons. There are two products required for this cleanse: Bulking Agent and Herbal Enhancement Formula. These can be purchased at most health food stores.
* WORK ON PSYCHOSPIRITUAL ISSUES:
  SMALL INTESTINE: ability to take in and absorb and assimilate all aspects of our lives
  COLON: ability to let go of that which no longer serves us

Liver and gallbladder

* Eat the highest quality food possible, emphasizing 80% fruit and vegetables.
* Decrease all fats in general and eliminate processed fats.
* Improve digestion by following the guidelines outlined in this book.
* WORK ON PSYCHOSPIRITUAL ISSUES:
  LIVER: ability to process and express anger in healthy ways
  GALLBLADDER: ability to let go of bitterness and the past.

Urinary system

* Decrease or eliminate processed foods, poor quality fats, salt and salty condiments, high protein foods (flesh, dairy and eggs).
* Drink the purest water available. Pure spring water is best. Otherwise drink reverse osmosis or distilled water. It could be wise to rotate various types of water if you are not absolutely sure of the purity.
* WORK ON PSYCHOSPIRITUAL ISSUES:
  KIDNEYS: ability to process fear and other negative emotions, to let them flow through us retaining only the lessons
  BLADDER: ability to let go of negative emotions, to not let ourselves get irritated, fearful, and anxious

Respiratory system

"Seek the fresh air of the forest and of the fields, and there in the midst of them shall you find the angel of air... I tell you truly, the angel of air shall cast out of your body all uncleanness which defiled it without and within." EGP 1

* Be aware of proper breathing and practice breathwork (pranayam).
* Spend time in nature.
* Sleep with the window slightly open, or better yet outdoors.
* Plant indoor and outdoor plants and trees.
* Generally avoid or reduce mucus forming foods (especially dairy and wheat).
* Do daily movement that you enjoy.
* Avoid chemical cleaners in the home.
* Use herbal steams (eucalyptus, thyme, oregano).
* Install air filters.
* Use a nedi pot to clean your sinuses.
* WORK ON PSYCHOSPIRITUAL ISSUES:
  LUNGS: ability to take in life, to allow oneself to be inspired
  SINUSES: ability to enjoy and accept life as it is, in the moment

Skin and lymphatic system

* Expose your skin to gentle sunlight.

"Put off your shoes and your clothing and suffer the angel of sunlight to embrace all your body. Then breathe long and deep, that the angel of sunlight may be brought within you." EGP 1

* Shower in lukewarm or cold water, morning and evening. Try finishing off all showers with as cold water as possible for as long as possible. This will close your pores, bring blood to the surface, increase circulation, tighten skin, and leave you feeling invigorated.

"I tell you truly, the angel of water shall cast out of your body all uncleanness which defiled it without and within." EGP 1

* Use only natural skin creams and cosmetics with natural ingredients.
* Do daily movement and exercise.
* Be aware of proper breathing and practice breathwork (pranayam).
* Get a massage.
* Dry brush your skin.
* Take saunas and steam baths.
* BATHS:
    Epsom salts: helps eliminate toxins by activating fluid movement in the tissues and increasing perspiration – start with 1/2 cup and increase to 4 cups, soak for 20 minutes and rinse body well after.
    Sea salt: detoxifies radiation – up to 1/2 kg per tub.
    Baking soda: makes body more alkaline – 1/4 kg per tub.
    Cider vinegar: normalizes skin pH – 1/2 to 1 cup per tub.
* WORK ON PSYCHOSPIRITUAL ISSUES:
    SKIN: ability to feel safe being authentic
    LYMPHATICS: ability to allow oneself to be fully alive as a physical being.

"Your Mother is in you, and you in her. She bore you: she gives you life. It was she who gave to you your body, and to her shall you one day give it back. Happy are you when you come to know her and her kingdom; if you receive your Mother's angels and if you do her laws. I tell you truly, he who does these things shall never see disease. For the power of our Mother is above all."
THE ESSENE GOSPEL OF PEACE

"Behold,

I have given you every herb bearing seed,

which is upon the face of all the earth,

and every tree, in which is the fruit of a

tree yielding seed;

to you it shall be for meat...

but flesh and the blood which quickens it,

shall ye not eat."

THE ESSENE GOSPEL OF PEACE

Vegetarianism

"Nothing will benefit human health and increase the chances for survival of life on earth as the evolution to a vegetarian diet." ALBERT EINSTEIN

OUR CURRENT ANIMAL-PRODUCT CENTERED NORTH AMERICAN DIET HAS FAR-REACHING AND OFTEN DEVASTATING EFFECTS ON OUR FELLOW LIVING CREATURES, OUR HEALTH, AND OUR ENVIRONMENT.

"The time will come when men such as I will look upon the murder of animals as they now look upon the murder of men." LEONARDO DA VINCI

"You have just dined, and however scrupulously the slaughterhouse is concealed in the distance of miles, there is complicity." RALPH WALDO EMERSON

"It ill becomes us to invoke in our daily prayers the blessings of God, the compassionate, if we in turn will not practice elementary compassion towards our fellow creatures." MAHATMA GANDHI

Can they suffer?

In order to supply meat and animal products at the rate of North American consumption, most animals are raised on factory farms to maximize efficiency and profits. Very little, if any, attention is given to the fact that animals are sensitive creatures with complex behavioural patterns and are capable of suffering. They are raised in cramped, unsuitable conditions, are fed as cheaply as possible, are routinely given antibiotics and hormones, and exposed to pesticides. They are taken from their mothers at birth, de-beaked, tail-docked, kept in the dark. Many never see the light of day. They are stacked on top of each other, transported inside trucks in scorching heat and freezing cold, and lined up to be slaughtered, feeling the terror as they smell and sense their impending death. There are so many horrors going on daily in the meat industry as well as the dairy and egg industries—they are hard to see, to write about, and to hear about. When I first read about their lives I was deeply saddened and no longer wanted to be a part of it. (For more information go to www.meetyourmeat.com.)

This is health?

I had always rationalized my consumption of animal products by the fact that these foods contribute greatly to our health and well-being. The Four Food Groups approach to eating, which is taught in our schools, colleges, and universities and continues to be shared by medical professionals, perpetuates the myth regarding the necessity to consume animal products to be healthy. In fact, there is much recent research presented in reputable and respected scientific publications implicating excess animal product consumption in many of the degenerative diseases that plague our nation.

The human anatomy and physiology is that of a natural vegetarian and is vastly different from that of a natural carnivore. Vegetarians have fingers for gathering, flat teeth and a jaw structured for grinding fruit and vegetables, a long convoluted digestive system, digestive enzymes designed to break down complex carbohydrates, and a liver that can only process and excrete limited amounts of cholesterol (the rest of which is deposited in our tissues).

Many studies have shown that people who consume low-fat, high-fiber, vegetarian diets live longer and have lower cholesterol levels. They also suffer significantly less from heart attacks, many forms of cancer (breast, colon, prostate, ovarian, intestinal, etc.), high blood pressure, diabetes, osteoporosis, arthritis, kidney disease, kidney stones, gall stones, obesity, diverticulosis, ulcers, multiple sclerosis, and constipation. These diseases do not have to be an accepted element in our society. Much too much time and money is being spent on the research of treatment and medication when the real solution lies in prevention through a healthy lifestyle.

Realize that nutritional needs can easily be met on a pure vegetarian diet. Recent studies have shown that a whole foods vegetarian diet with sufficient calories has all the nutrients, including protein, that we need. Contrary to what you may believe, protein only needs to contribute 5 to 15 per cent to our caloric intake—excess protein intake has been directly linked to various forms of cancer, kidney disease, and osteoporosis (excess protein draws calcium out of the bones). A diet that draws from the major groups of fruit, vegetables, whole grains, legumes, nuts and seeds is fully health-supporting. On a personal note regarding health, both of my children have been raised from birth on vegetarian diets—they have never needed to take any drugs—not Tylenol, not aspirin, not antibiotics. On the rare occasions when they do get sick, it passes quickly. They are both elite athletes and excellent students.

Another important issue that I feel must be addressed is the fact that many of us are concerned, and with good reason, about ingesting pesticides (chlorinated hydrocarbons such as DDT and chlordane) and industrial wastes (such as PCBs and dioxin) in our diets. Much of the toxic residues that enter our bodies come from non-organic (primarily) meat, eggs, and dairy products. These toxins are fat-soluble substances that accumulate in the muscle tissue, fat, and milk of animals—these same animals are then made into your beef, pork, fish, poultry, and dairy products.

Here are some of the dynamic doctors who are advancing healthy vegetarian nutrition through their studies and work: Dr. T. Colin Campbell, www.thechinastudy.com; Dr. John McDougall, www.drmcdougall.com; Dr. Neal Barnard, www.nealbarnard.org; Dr. Michael Klaper, www.vegsource.com/klaper.

The most important environmental contribution that you can make

We are all aware of the worsening condition of our planet and many of us are trying to do what we can to help. As I read books, such as Diet for a New America, I was shocked to discover that North America's meat-centered diet has an extremely detrimental effect on the environment.

CONSIDER THESE FACTS:

* 40 times more fossil fuels are needed to produce a meat-centered diet. The primary cause of the greenhouse effect (global warming) is carbon dioxide emissions from fossil fuels.
* The world's known oil reserves would last 13 years if every human ate a meat-centered diet. They would last 260 years if humans no longer ate meat.
* 75% of the topsoil that was once here is gone, and 85% of this loss is directly related to livestock raising.
* The tropical rain forests are being cleared at astounding rates, mainly for cattle growing. The rain forests are important because they absorb carbon dioxide and therefore cut down on the greenhouse effect. Rain forests are also important as they are the home of many native tribes and animal and plant species (1,000 species per year become extinct as a result of deforestation). After 3 years, the cleared land is barren and useless, and more trees must be cleared to feed the cattle whose flesh is exported to Canada and the United States.
* It takes 25 gallons of water to produce one pound of wheat, 2,500 gallons to produce one pound of beef. Half of all the fresh water in North America goes towards meat production.
* The number one source of organic water pollution in North America is animal manure.
* Any given acreage can feed 20 times more people who are on a pure vegetarian diet than on a meat-centered diet. A change in North American diet would free up land for the planting of much-needed trees—trees that can absorb carbon dioxide, provide us with oxygen, stabilize the topsoil, and provide habitat for animal life.
* 20,000 pounds of potatoes can be grown on one acre, but only 165 pounds of beef can be grown on the same acre.
* 60 million people die of starvation every year. If North Americans were to reduce their intake of meat by only 10%, the animal feed grains that would be saved could adequately feed all of those people.

There are many other fascinating facts that are available through vegetarian groups and publications. In short, all things considered, our meat-centered diet is the number one eco-destructive force in North America today. For more information on the environmental implications of our food choices, and practical suggestions on what you can do, check out www.earthsave.com.

So what do we do with this information? Most of us know, on some level, that we humans have reached a crucial point in our evolution and existence on this planet. Time is in fact short. We are determining the fate of our beloved Earth with every choice that we make, from the cars that we drive, to the household cleaners that we use, and to what we put on our plates. Intention is crucial—if we look in our hearts, I suspect that we will all find a yearning for a cleaner, more peaceful, and more humane world. Owning this deep-seated desire is the key to slowly but surely beginning to make more and more choices to support the kind of world that we wish to live in. Sometimes when we think of the magnitude of the task at hand, we get overwhelmed and then shut down. There is so much to do, there are so many changes to make, and our lives are already so full. Breathe, be calm, and make one choice at a time. Even the small choices ultimately make a big difference. Don't expect to be perfect, and be gentle with yourself when you fall short of whatever so-called ideal you have set for yourself. Just do your best. When making choices, break automatic patterns and reflect with your heart and your head—use your wisdom and your love ... one choice at a time. Involve your family in the process.

Can you begin to incorporate more plant-based meals into your weeks? How can you alter your favourite recipes to contain less, fewer, or no animal products? Can you try one or two new vegetarian recipes every week? Are you ready to enjoy all of the various kinds of exciting and delicious vegetarian ethnic dishes that are available?

"Blessed is the Child of light who is strong in body, for he shall have oneness with the Earth.... he who hath found peace with the body hath built a holy temple wherein may dwell forever the Spirit of God." ESSENE GOSPEL OF PEACE, BOOK 2

"But I do say to you:
Kill neither men, nor beasts,
nor yet the food which goes into your mouth.
For if you eat living food,
the same food will quicken you,
but if you kill your food,
the dead food will kill you also.
For life comes only from life,
and from death comes always death.
For everything which kills your food,
kills your bodies also.
And everything which kills your bodies
kills your souls also.
And your bodies become what your foods are,
even as your spirits, likewise,
become what your thoughts are.
Therefore eat not anything
which fire, or frost, or water has destroyed.
For burned, frozen and rotten foods
will burn, freeze and rot
your bodies also."

THE ESSENE GOSPEL OF PEACE

Living Foods

I believe that the nutritional trend that will carry us through into a time of health and peace on this Earth will include not only a vegetarian diet but also a diet that includes more and more live, uncooked foods. Humans and their domesticated animals are the only species that cook their foods—they are also plagued with the most physical, mental, and emotional distress. The more my respect for nature and her laws deepens, the more I trust her wisdom. The food that has been provided for us by nature is perfect: balanced, nutrient-rich, and alive. More and more people are realizing the incredible power of living foods by adopting more living foods diets and enjoying tremendous health and life benefits.

What are living foods?

Living foods are foods that are eaten in their natural state and are not cooked (not heated above 118F). Vegetables, fruit, nuts, seeds, grains, and sometimes dairy products are eaten in their raw state. There is a whole cuisine evolving around this concept, and many books outlining the philosophy and the science behind raw foods, as well as recipe books, are being made available to us. Also, many health professionals following live foods diets are providing shining and inspirational examples of health to us. Gabriel Cousens, Victoria Boutenko and her family, Ann Wigmore, Brian Clement, David Wolfe, and Storm and Jinjee Talifero are just some examples of modern day live foods pioneers.

Reasons to eat more raw

THERE ARE MANY REASONS TO INCORPORATE MORE LIVE FOODS INTO YOUR DIET.

* As mentioned above, humans are the only species to cook their food and we suffer from the most degenerative diseases.

* The life force of any food, measured by the intensity of the electromagnetic or energy field captured through Kirlian photography, decreases as we cook foods. (Check out www.kirlian.com for pictures.) Consider this ... plant two sunflower seeds: one raw, one toasted. Which one will grow? Which one is alive? Which one, when eaten, will impart more aliveness to your body based on the universal energy field principle of harmonic inductance?

* Living water, contained in living foods, has a unique energy and configuration which looks like frozen snowflake crystals observed under a high-powered micro scope. When foods are cooked, the form of the water changes and is quite obviously less alive and vibrant. Cooking has a deadening effect on the water contained in foods.

* Heating foods above 118F destroys enzymes. Food enzymes are in every raw food. The types of enzymes are specific to the type of food. An avocado will

contain high amounts of fat-digesting enzymes because of its high fat content, whereas an apple will contain proportionately larger amounts of carbohydrate-digesting enzymes because of its high carbohydrate content. Once we cook that apple though, say to make apple sauce, the enzymes are destroyed and our bodies will have to compensate by secreting more from all of the digestive organs (especially the pancreas). If we are constantly eating large quantities of cooked foods, the immune system will provide back-up by sending white blood cells to lend some of their enzymes to break down the food. This is called digestive leukocytosis. This back-up system is helpful in the short term, but in the long term it weakens the immune system by diverting its efforts towards digestion rather than identifying and destroying cancer cells, bacteria, viruses, and other invaders.

✳ In the Pottenger's Cats Study performed between 1932 and 1942, one group of cats was fed predominantly raw foods while the other group was fed cooked foods. The group fed cooked foods showed signs of decreased reproductive capacity, organ malfunctions, and skeletal deformities which worsened with each generation. I'll share my own experience with Crystal, my Chinese Shar-pei. These dogs, also commonly known as wrinkle dogs, typically suffer from ill-health in the form of skin disorders, fevers, kidney disease, and joint inflammation. I put Crystal on a raw foods diet after noticing that she was experiencing skin problems, cloudy eyes, sore joints, and fevers. She eats raw ground up vegetables, raw chicken bones and meat, and organs and is doing well. After about two years on this diet and initial detoxification symptoms, her coat is beautiful, she scratches far less, no longer suffers from sore joints and fever, and her eyes are clearer. At 10-years-old, she looks and acts like a much younger dog. Do a search under "BARF diet" (Biologically Appropriate Raw Foods) to find many helpful links on raw diets for dogs and cats.

✳ Whenever food is cooked, many of the original nutrients are altered, often with harmful effects: proteins coagulate making them more difficult to absorb, overheated fats generate numerous carcinogens, natural fiber breaks down and loses its ability to sweep the intestines clean, 30 to 50 per cent of vitamins are destroyed, pesticides are restructured into even more toxic compounds, oxygen is lost, etc. For more information on these changes and more, visit www.living-foods.com.

✳ Also my web site www.carolinedupont.com has many links to raw foods web sites.

GENERALLY IT IS ADVISABLE TO GRADUALLY INCREASE YOUR INTAKE OF LIVING FOODS OVER TIME. THE TOTAL PERCENTAGE OF RAW ADVISABLE DEPENDS ON HEALTH CONDITIONS, CURRENT HABITS, SEASON OF THE YEAR, EMOTIONAL STATE, SPIRITUAL AWARENESS, AND INTERNAL READINESS. FOR MOST PEOPLE, 30 TO 80 PER CENT WOULD BE IDEAL TO START.

How to incorporate more live foods into your diet

* Eat more fresh raw fruit and vegetables
* Make meals of fruit, fruit salads, and fruit smoothies
* Expand the variety of fruit and vegetables that you consume
* Eat at least one type of raw food at each meal
* Have a large salad every day
* Drink fresh-pressed raw vegetable juices
* Buy a raw foods cookbook
* Attend a live foods education/preparation class
* Try some of the live foods recipes in this book
* Support your living foods diet with a steady spiritual practice

"I have reached the inner vision and through Thy spirit in me I have heard Thy wondrous secret. Through Thy mystic insight Thou hast caused a spring of knowledge to well up within me, a fountain of power pouring forth living waters, a flood of love and all embracing wisdom like the splendor of eternal Light." FROM "THE BOOK OF HYMNS" OF THE DEAD SEA SCROLLS

Prayer for Health:
Dear God,
As I rise up today,
I thank You for the opportunity to be on this Earth
in these powerful times.
I thank You for my body. I thank You for my life.
Please bless my entire being and use it for Your purposes.
May I make choices that nurture my body
so that I may best serve You.
Be in my hands when I prepare and eat
the health-giving food
that You so graciously provide for me through
this precious Earth.
Be in my head when I make choices as I fill my days,
that they may bring me closer to perfect health
and closer to You.
Be in my heart always so that all that I give
in my thoughts, my words, my work and my deeds
contributes to my health and to the health of this world.
May I rise up strong today, and may my body and soul
radiate Your love and Your beauty.
Purify my mind, my heart, my body.
May every cell of my being be filled with Your light.
May both my body and soul be illumined
for Your sake and for the sake of all the world.
Amen.

INSPIRED BY PRAYERS BY MARIANNE WILLIAMSON IN
ILLUMINATA: A RETURN TO PRAYER

Rob's Story

Rob came to me as a client after attending a meditation class and finding out that I was a holistic health practitioner. He had been facing some serious health challenges for quite a while due to poor lifestyle and in part to having been born 3 1/2 weeks early which caused all of his organs to under-function. He had just been hospitalized with severe pancreatitis, had been suffering from colitis for 25 years, and had gallstones and liver disease. He was told that he would need a liver transplant in 10 years. He was on sleep medication and was 50 pounds overweight. We found out that a mutual friend had told him to see me months before but he had lost the e-mail and never followed up. Anyway, here was his second opportunity and he took it. As he sat down in my healing room, he looked me in the eye and very earnestly proclaimed that I should know that he was putting his complete trust in me and that he would follow everything that I told him to do. I prescribed a diet made up mainly of fruit and vegetables (mostly cooked at the beginning but eventually we added more and more raw), plus minimal amounts of non-glutenous grains like brown rice and quinoa. Every week we would go into my kitchen and prepare a vegetable soup or a smoothie which he would take home. As he had promised, he followed the diet perfectly and began to feel much better. I also did ongoing energy work on him to help release the psychospiritual issues that were the root cause of his physical symptoms. He continued with regular meditation and yoga.

I have received many gifts from my relationship with Rob. Beyond the gift of a man with a heart of gold, I have witnessed first-hand the miracle of healing. Although I have felt the blessing of physical energy, and mental, emotional, and spiritual clarity that come with a healthy lifestyle, I myself have never had any serious health problems. The extent of Rob's healing has been tremendous. After 4 months on his new program he had lost 30 pounds and was no longer on any medication. He had passed all of his gallstones, and his colitis was under control. He had his liver counts tested and his doctor was so surprised that they were normal that he had him re-tested! Again they were normal. As an open-minded physician, he cautiously encouraged him to continue doing what he was doing. So, after suffering from poor health much of his life, he is well on his way to good health.

Yes, health problems can be reversed with proper diet, meditation, yoga, emotional work, and other choices, not the least of which is love...

On the Process of Transformation

Soon after I began giving talks about nutrition and health, I became fascinated with the process of human change. Many of us have the information we need to move us forward in ways that we obviously desire, but often we aren't able to take this information and consistently incorporate it into our lives. This has been as frustrating for me as a human being, and as a health professional, as it no doubt is for you! I have learned from my own experience that good intentions are not always enough. What are the mental and emotional reasons behind a resistance to effortlessly taking care of ourselves on a consistent basis? How does information move from the brain into the body? I hope that the following reflections and suggestions will help you to create the health that you dream of.

HEALTH IS A CONSCIOUS CHOICE THAT TAKES SELF-RESPONSIBILITY, LOVE, COMMITMENT, COURAGE, AND GENTLENESS.

There are a few key words here. "CONSCIOUS" means that we are aware of the choices that we make and that our choices are internally driven. That is, we listen to our own inner signals rather than to what we see around us in advertisements or the latest fad diet book.

We make our choices from a place of SELF-RESPONSIBILITY—unless we are babies, we are the ones who are making our food choices on a meal-to-meal basis. We often want to blame genetics, stress, relationships, and circumstances for the way that we eat, look, and feel. The truth is that each one of us is ultimately responsible for our food choices, our health, and our quality of life.

The most important form of love is SELF-LOVE. Eating excellent quality food is a love letter to yourself. The gift of self-love is that we will be able to love others more unconditionally. And the more we give, the more we receive. What foods do you eat when you love yourself?

COMMITMENT maintains our focus and assures our success in any venture.

COURAGE is what is needed to change, to grow and to eat differently than others.

GENTLENESS with ourselves is needed because taking responsibility for our health is a process that often involves regressing and not living up to our standards. This is normal. Continue to be aware, learn the lesson inherent in every challenge rather than berating yourself with guilt and judgment, and move on.

Accept where you are today

No matter where you're starting, no matter what your health challenge, no matter what your current diet, the only place to begin is where you are now. Forgive yourself for not loving yourself fully in the past and begin now. Pray for assistance.

You will know when you are ready for change

On the one hand, health changes require discipline. On the other hand, a large component of success in these health ventures is a certain internal ripeness. Continue to listen for and to heed internal signals, and make changes at a pace that feels comfortable for you. Some people make huge shifts overnight, some go in spurts, and others make tiny additions. We are all different people, living different circumstances, with varying paths to the same ultimate goal.

However, if you have a serious health problem you have to be swift, focused, and disciplined in your approach to healing. The longer a disease has progressed, the more intense the healing plan will have to be. Ask for help and direction from holistic health professionals.

Read literature, attend courses, surround yourself with people who will reinforce the changes you are making with respect to your health

Surround yourself with positive influences. You will naturally draw these to you as you commit to your health.

Notice when you are eating to satisfy emotional needs and ask yourself how you could fill those needs in another way

Emotions will be your greatest challenge on this path to health. So much of what goes into our mouths is emotionally driven. Know this, be a witness to this, feel your emotions deeply, retain the wisdom, get some help. Keep a journal. Make meditation a daily commitment. Awareness through meditation is the most powerful practice that I know of for releasing emotions and patterns that no longer serve us. It balances the brain and the nervous system, the endocrine system, and the immune system.

Set your intention to experience eating as a ritual to feed your body and nourish your soul

When you get your soul involved in any venture, success is guaranteed! It's the place in your being that is already perfect and it will not steer you wrong.

Respect other people's right to make their own choices

Many times when we begin to make changes we want to convert everyone around us. This seems to come from genuine caring, but in reality arises from insecurity and a need to be supported by outside sources. The more you listen to your own inner voice, the less you will need outside approval. Also, we all want the freedom to make our own choices when we are ready. Truly, no one wants to be told what to do, much less what to eat. If you want others to respect your food choices, then respect theirs.

Also, the best way to affect others is to live your ideals as best you can and to reflect vitality, health, and humility. As Gandhi said: "Be the change that you want to see in the world".

Add good foods to your daily choices – gradually they will crowd out bad foods

Psychologically this makes sense. Anytime something is taken away from you, you want it more. So start introducing yourself to new, healthy, delicious foods. You can only eat so much. As you look back, you will see that you eat far less of the unhealthy foods that you used to eat and you don't even miss them.

Stock your home with only healthy foods

No matter how disciplined you are, when there's junk food around, you and your family will be tempted, especially at first when you still have emotional attachments to them. Keep them out of the house, perhaps treat yourself to them when you're out (and enjoy them guilt-free in these cases).

Lovingly explain to your family what you are doing and why

If you are doing the food shopping and preparation, you will need to involve your family in the process that you are going through. You may have a mutiny on your hands if all of the sudden their favourite so-called foods are not readily available at home. Every family will have to work out its own solution and reach a peaceful compromise. I think it helps to share new information that you are learning about health and nutrition (to the extent that your family is able to absorb it), and don't be afraid to show your passion, inspiration, and desire for health for yourself and them.

Listen to the expert inside – use your intuition, your mind, and your heart

Any health information needs to be filtered through your logical mind, your feeling heart, and your intuitive body. Use these personal tools to joyfully and creatively create a nutritional approach that works for you. Remain as aware as possible every step of the way.

*"Never underestimate the impact of single individuals, working sincerely
to create health, understanding, and peace in their own lives.
For every step we take to establish genuinely healthy food choices
is a step into our own wholeness, into the power to create healthy lives
for ourselves, and to contribute to the health and well-being of others.
... Every time we say 'yes' to foods that nourish our bodies and spirits,
and every time we say 'no' to foods that aren't good for us
we are saying 'yes' to life.
We are afforded an extraordinary opportunity today.
By choosing to eat more healthfully and more consciously,
we can take a stand on behalf of ourselves
and our interconnectedness with the rest of humanity.
At a personal level we may be simply saying that we do not want to
cause ourselves to suffer a heart attack.
But at the same time we can add our voice to the mounting chorus
calling for a world in which our land, our water, our energy,
and our labor are used to grow food for people to eat
rather than feed our livestock.
We do not yet know what it would be like
to live in a truly healthy and compassionate society.
But there are some things that are available to us now:
We can know the fulfillment of working toward such a world.
We can know the liberation of freeing ourselves from habits
that are not natural and do not serve us,
but have come to pass for normal in our society.
We can know the power of uniting with others in working
to bring understanding and clarity where it is so greatly needed.
May all be fed, May all be healed, May all be loved."*

JOHN ROBBINS IN MAY ALL BE FED

Making Changes:
Practical Advice on How to Start

In Natural Life magazine, writer Lorna Sass says:

"Cooking takes time, and at some point I just surrendered to that fact. What a relief! It took the threat of surgery to finally understand that it makes no sense whatsoever to give short shrift to one of life's most nourishing activities.

By making meal preparation a high priority on my daily 'to do' list, it became easier to complete the job without resentment or rushing. This leisurely approach gradually awakened a new respect for Nature's bounty and for Earth itself!"

No doubt, you will find at first that your improved eating habits require more preparation time. In my experience, once you discover new stores, fill your cupboards with staples, acquire a repertoire of favourite quick recipes, and get adjusted to your new routine, you will find that time spent in the kitchen will decrease. It does take more time to prepare a typical meal consisting of food made from fresh whole ingredients than it does to rely on processed packaged foods. The goal is to make you feel healthy and whole (not stressed out!). So here are some suggestions that I hope will help you:

* Have a family meeting. Discuss the changes you would like to make and why. Ask for everybody's input on the strategy for implementation and arrive at a peaceful compromise.

* For the first little while it helps to sit down and plan the menu for the week in advance. Choose foods and recipes that are relatively familiar to your family and keep it simple.

* From recipes, make a shopping list. Keep a running list on your kitchen counter of items that you need at the grocery store, the health food store, and/or the market. Add to the list as soon as you run out of the particular item. Note: at first you may find yourself buying more than you are accustomed to because you are stocking your shelves with the ingredients necessary for whole foods cooking. Once you are stocked up, you'll be buying and spending less.

* Create a relaxing atmosphere during food preparation: set aside the time that you need and let your family know that during this time they are basically on their own (spouse can be with kids, or they can sit at the table and do homework or crafts, or help out with some of the food preparation, etc.); make sure that your kitchen is organized; buy good quality appliances and cooking utensils; put on some pleasant music, sing, meditate, be with yourself.

* Keep your meals simple.

* Do as much advanced preparation as possible, especially if you come home from work close to dinnertime.

* Keep your home stocked with fresh fruit (most of these can be piled attractively into baskets on your counter) and vegetables; your freezer with nuts, seeds, whole grain breads, and some healthy convenience foods; your cupboards with canned legumes, whole grains, pastas, and jarred sauces.

* Organize your kitchen, keeping it simple, clean, and inviting. Put similar items in the same cupboard (for example: nuts, seeds, dried fruit, dried legumes and grains, pastas, cereals, spices, crackers, cans, etc.).

* Keep dried fruit, nuts, seeds, grains, flours, dry legumes, etc. in labeled glass jars preferably (or good quality stable plastic containers) so that they stay fresh and are easy to find and organize.

* Stock your kitchen with whole foods snacks only: fresh fruit and vegetables, nuts, dried fruit, whole grain breads, crackers and muffins, wholesome cookies. Your family will get used to not having unhealthy snacks around.

* I have found it helpful to always have a big pot of hearty soup prepared. Store it in the refrigerator for up to 4 days. This makes a great lunch or dinner with a salad, or even a snack. If you pack your lunches, put some in a thermos for a warm meal away from home.

* Always have at least one spread or filling for wraps, sandwiches, or pita pockets on hand. We like avocado, nut and seed pâtés, hummus, baba ganoush, tofu spread, organic cheese.

* Although not ideal nutritionally, it is helpful and practical to double recipes for leftovers the next day or to freeze for some day in the future when you want to take a break from cooking.

* Serve a wide variety of foods throughout the week. Ask your family to be open to trying new dishes. Don't expect them to be delighted with every new concoction that you create. Apparently a child has to taste a new food at least 11 times before accepting it as a part of his/her repertoire. Maybe the same goes for adults!

* Be patient with yourself and your family—the changes you're making, although positive, can still be stressful. Keep motivated by sharing with friends who have the same interest in healthy eating. Go to your local library and borrow books on nutrition and food preparation that reflect and support your new choices.

* Set your intention on a long-term goal of radiant health for you and your family.

"On the joy of discovery:
There are times when a sense of urgency spurs us on
to probe and question and overturn what has been,
so that new growth can be brought into being.
And there are times when we feel
that we have all the time we could possibly need to grow into ourselves.
But once we experience the immense satisfaction
that comes when we uncover a shadowed area of our life
and bring it into the light, we are changed forever
and something essential to our quest is quickened.
For when we taste the freedom
that comes from liberating our life force from fear and stagnation,
we are never again quite as willing
to return to a life of unconscious action."

JOHN ROBBINS AND ANN MORTIFEE

Dietary Transitions

"... so just take whatever steps seem easiest for you, and as you take a few steps it will become easier for you to take a few more ..." PEACE PILGRIM IN STEPS TOWARDS INNER PEACE

The following are transition guidelines for people who have no major health problems. The sequence given is simply a suggestion and your own transformation will take on its own pattern. If you do have serious symptoms, please consult a health practitioner and/or a holistic nutritionist for specific recommendations. In this case you will have to make more drastic changes.

I have seen that the general pattern for most successful health aspirants is the same. First there is an increased consumption of natural foods, including organic. Also, the intake of fruit and vegetables increases and the intake of animal products decreases. Overall, the relative proportion of raw and living foods increases as time passes.

Idea

TO TRANSITION TO A NEW STAGE IN YOUR EATING HABITS, DO WHATEVER YOU ARE ASPIRING TO DO ONE DAY A WEEK. SO IF YOU ARE TRYING TO EAT LESS DAIRY OR WHEAT, CHOOSE AT LEAST ONE DAY A WEEK WHERE YOU EAT NONE AT ALL. OR IF YOU WANT TO EAT MORE LIVING FOODS, CHOOSE ONE DAY TO EAT ONLY RAW FOODS. THIS WILL CAUSE YOU TO NATURALLY LOOK FOR ALTERNATIVES AND BEFORE YOU KNOW IT THE QUANTITIES OF THESE FOODS WILL CHANGE EFFORTLESSLY. AND YOU WILL BEGIN TO EXPERIENCE AND ENJOY FIRST-HAND THE BENEFITS OF MAKING THESE CHANGES.

In all of the following stages, gradually progress to as many organic, bio-dynamic, heritage, and wild choices as possible.

Beverages

Stage 1
* limit coffee and tea – substitute herbal beverages
* limit alcohol and carbonated beverages – substitute natural soft drinks
* increase pure fruit and vegetable juices
* introduce freshly made fruit and vegetable juices
  (you will need to purchase a juicer to do this)
* eliminate tap water – use distilled, reverse osmosis, or spring water
Stage 2
* eliminate caffeinated beverages
* limit natural soft drinks
* limit store-bought pasteurized fruit and vegetable juices
* drink fresh pressed juice (preferably green)
Stage 3
* drink only purified water, herbal teas, and fresh pressed juices

Carbohydrates

Stage 1
* use whole grain breads (no added chemicals)
* explore breads made from a variety of grains: kamut, spelt, rye, barley, etc.
Stage 2
* introduce breads made from sprouted grains
Stage 3
* use only sprouted and/or raw breads and crackers and Essene breads

CEREALS:

Stage 1
* use only whole grain cereals without additives or preservatives
Stage 2
* use cooked whole grains for your morning cereal (oatmeal, rice, kasha, etc.)
Stage 3
* use whole, raw, sprouted grains (uncooked)

GRAINS:

Stages 1
* expand the variety of grains used: try brown rice, quinoa, millet, barley
Stage 2
* use whole gluten-free grains most often:
    brown rice (long-grain, short-grain, basmati, jasmine, etc.),
    quinoa, millet, buckwheat, amaranth
Stage 3
* decrease consumption of all grains

PASTAS:

Stage 1
* minimize white flour pastas
* introduce rice, kamut, buckwheat, whole wheat pastas
Stages 2 and 3
* decrease the use of pasta
* use a spiral slicer to create vegetable 'pasta'

Sweeteners

Stage 1
* eliminate white sugar
* eliminate chemical sweeteners: aspartame, nutrasweet, saccharin
* use dark brown sugar, sucanat, honey, maple syrup, rice syrup, barley malt, unsulphured molasses

Stage 2
* use raw honey, maple syrup, agave syrup, sucanat in limited quantities

Stage 3
* limit or eliminate use of natural sweeteners

Fruit

Stage 1
* increase intake of fresh fruit, emphasizing local fruit
* limit canned fruit (packed in their own juice)
* increase use of unsulphured dried fruit that has been reconstituted with water

Stages 2 and 3
* use only fresh tree-ripened fruit
* limit use of hybridized or seedless fruit

Desserts and sweets

Stage 1
* cut back on desserts by half
* choose desserts made from fresh wholesome ingredients

Stage 2
* limit store-bought desserts and sweets, even natural ones
* eliminate desserts following meals

Stage 3
* use as snack only
* make from fresh raw ingredients only (raw fruit pies with nut crusts, raw fruit and nut cookies and candies, whole fruit smoothies or ice cream)

Fats and oils

EXTRACTED OILS:

Stage 1
* eliminate margarine
* limit use of refined oils
* use cold pressed vegetable oils (flax, hemp, olive, coconut, sesame, etc.)
* use raw unsalted butter in limited quantities

Stage 2

* further reduce intake of butter
* use only cold pressed oils in dark bottles

Stage 3

* eliminate butter
* reduce use of cold pressed oils

Stage 1

* use unsalted nuts and seeds
* limit intake of non-organic peanut butters
* increase intake of raw nuts and seeds (soaked when possible)

Stage 2

* limit intake of nut butters
* limit intake of roasted nuts and seeds

Stage 3

* use only raw or soaked nuts and seeds
* use only raw nut butters

Proteins

Stage 1

* limit use of all dairy (especially milk and non-organic cheeses)
* use raw goat-milk products
* use soy, rice, grain, and almond milks more often

Stage 2

* use organic, raw, un-homogenized dairy more often
* use freshly made nut milks more often

Stage 3

* limit use of dairy or eliminate dairy

Stage 1

* limit use

Stage 2

* use organic, free-range, fertile eggs

Stage 3

* limit use further, or eliminate eggs

Vegetables

Stage 1

* increase quantity of vegetables consumed
* use organic more often
* choose fresh over frozen and canned
* explore new vegetables – particularly green leafy and root vegetables. Try kale, collards, swiss chard, bok choy, arugula, spinach, green cabbage, parsnips, yams, celery root, beets, turnips, squash, etc.
* use a wider variety of colours
* add sprouts (sunflower, alfalfa, red clover, lentil, radish, onion, etc.) to your daily selections

Stage 2

* increase raw vegetables
* continue to add new vegetables to your daily selections
* consume at least one large green salad every day

Stage 3

* consider eating most of your vegetables live and raw

Condiments and Seasonings

Stage 1

* explore natural versions of ketchup, mustard, mayonnaise, etc.
* replace soya sauce with tamari or Bragg's Liquid Seasoning
* begin to use only Celtic or Normandy gray sea salt
* use herbs and spices to season food

Stages 2 and 3

* use non-irradiated or fresh herbs and spices
* decrease or eliminate use of salt

"Realization frees you from outside influences.
It makes you stand by yourself.
The only way to escape from all sins, to stand above all temptations,
is to realize the true self.
Stand on your own two feet whether you are great or small,
whether you are highly placed or otherwise...
Realize your Divinity and everything is done."

V.T. NEELAKANTAN
IN MYSTICISM UNLOCKED (OF KRIYA BABAJI)

However...

Many of the previous sections have focused on guiding you on what to eat, how to eat, and how to transition to a wholesome diet however ...

WHEN YOU FIND THAT:
* Your eating is 'out of control',
* You're eating beyond your physical hunger,
* You're eating emotionally,
* You're making food choices out of fear,
* You follow periods of 'good' eating with 'bad' choices,
* You're eating late at night,
* You're thinking about food all of the time;

It's time to let go of strict rules and to focus on the root of the issue which is no doubt a combination of mental, emotional and spiritual factors.

HERE ARE SOME AFFIRMATIONS WHICH WILL LEAD YOU TO GREATER INNER PEACE AND MORE BALANCED FOOD CHOICES:

* I am willing to change.
* I love and approve of myself.
* I eat what I want, when I want.
* I eat to satisfy my hunger.
* I eat without distractions (TV, phone, car, books, computer, etc.).
* I eat with awareness.
* I enjoy the beauty, smell, taste and feel of my food.
* I eat with reverence and grace.
* I eat to nourish my body and soul.
* I trust my body's wisdom to guide me to the best foods for me.
* I eat with true enjoyment and gusto.

Say these at least twice a day sensing within your body how it feels to live each affirmation. This is important. It's not enough to simply say the words. Living these affirmations is the only way to consistently make balanced choices and to heal. At first, because you are allowing yourself to eat 'what you want, when you want', you may find that you choose foods that you have been depriving yourself of. Trust that your body, if allowed, will eventually find its natural ability to make consistent nourishing choices. It's most helpful to say affirmations before meditation and then to repeat them again at the end. If needed, in addition to meditation and feeling-based intentions and affirmations, get some professional help working through the real issues. Working through food issues is a valuable process into your Self that can reap great rewards.

"You are given the gifts of the gods; You create your reality according to your beliefs. Yours is the creative energy that makes the world. There are no limitations to the self, except those you believe in." JANE ROBERTS AS SETH

Stocking Your Kitchen

Fruit and vegetables

* Fresh fruit in season, as well as some nutrition-packed tropical fruit like mango, pineapple, papaya, young coconuts, durian
* Fresh vegetables: lettuce (romaine, leaf, arugula, baby greens, etc.), celery, peppers, zucchini, yam, potato, carrot, beet, radish, squash, rutabaga, leek, onion, garlic, leafy greens, kale, Swiss chard, spinach, watercress, tomato, cabbage, broccoli, cauliflower, others in season
* Sprouts: sunflower, buckwheat, alfalfa, clover, etc.
* Frozen vegetables: peas, corn, leftovers from summer harvest
* Tomato sauce and tomato paste
* Avocados
* Lemons and limes
* Frozen berries from summer harvest
* Dried fruit: figs, dates, apricots, apples, currants, raisins, coconut, etc. (buy unsulphured and organic if possible)
* Raw olives

Whole grain products

* Ezekiel 4:9 sprouted grain wraps, breads, and cereals (find these at your health food store, mostly in the freezer)
* Essene and Manna bread
* Brown rice (long-grain, short-grain, basmati, jasmine, wild, etc.)
* Whole grains: barley, quinoa, millet, oats, bulgur, cornmeal, wheat berries, buckwheat, etc.
* Dry cereals (ideally they should contain no refined sugar, no preservatives, very little salt, and be made with organic, preferably sprouted, grains)
* Hot cereals for porridge
* Whole grain pastas: rice, whole wheat, kamut, spelt, buckwheat, etc.
* Whole grain flours: spelt, kamut, wheat
* Whole grain crackers
* Rice cakes
* Popcorn
* Baked corn chips
* Whole grain bread
* Pita bread

Beans and bean products

* Dried peas and beans: green and yellow split peas, kidney beans, black beans, chick peas, lentils, navy, white beans, etc.
* Canned beans
* Tofu (Chinese firm blocks and Japanese silken in aseptic packages)

Nuts, seeds, and butters

* Nuts: raw almonds, cashews, walnuts, pecans, Brazil nuts, macadamias, etc.
* Nut butters: almond, cashew, peanut
* Seeds: sunflower, pumpkin, hemp, sesame, flax, poppy, etc.
* Seeds for sprouting: alfalfa, radish, red clover, lentils, etc.

Sweeteners

* Honey
* Sucanat
* Maple syrup
* Agave syrup
* Molasses
* Barley malt syrup
* Rice syrup

Dairy and substitutes

* Organic eggs
* Milk: organic dairy, soy, almond, or rice (Yu and Edensoy are good brands)
* Cheese: organic dairy, raw
* Yogourt and kefir (organic dairy)

Fats and oils

* Extra virgin olive oil
* Coconut oil
* Hemp seed oil
* Flax seed oil
* Organic butter and ghee
* Other cold-pressed oils: sunflower, walnut, sesame
* Combination cold pressed oils (for example: Udo's Choice and Essential Balance)

Seasonings and condiments

* Gray sea salt: Celtic or Normandy
* Pepper
* Dulse flakes
* Kelp powder
* Herbamare
* Tamari
* Bragg's Liquid Seasoning
* Fruit-sweetened ketchup
* Natural mustard
* Natural relish
* Natural salsa
* Natural mayonnaise
* Vegetable broth powder
* Vinegars: balsamic, apple cider, rice, red wine

Herbs and spices (these will give you a good start)

* Fresh herbs (you can grow these in your garden or your kitchen):
  parsley, basil, thyme, oregano, tarragon, cilantro, sage, etc.
* Dried herbs and spices (make sure you buy non-irradiated – Frontier and BioGO
  are good brands): allspice, basil, cayenne pepper/powder, celery seed, chili powder,
  cinnamon, ground cloves, coriander, cumin, curry, dill weed, ginger, mustard
  powder, nutmeg, oregano, paprika, parsley, rosemary, sage, tarragon, thyme,
  turmeric, etc.

Miscellaneous

* Nutritional yeast
* Seaweed (nori, kombu, arame, hijiki, dulse, etc.)
* Miso
* Arrowroot powder
* Vanilla
* Baking soda
* Baking powder

"Gratitude unlocks the fullness of life. It turns what we have into enough, and more. It turns denial into acceptance, chaos to order, confusion to clarity. It can turn a meal into a feast, a house into a home, a stranger into a friend. Gratitude makes sense of your past, brings peace for today, and creates a vision for tomorrow." MELODY BEATTIE

"Until one is committed there is hesitancy,
the chance to draw back, always ineffectiveness.
Concerning all acts of initiative and creation
there is one elementary truth,
the ignorance of which kills countless ideas and splendid plans:
that the moment one definitely commits oneself,
then providence moves too.
All sorts of things occur to help one
that would otherwise never have occurred.
A whole stream of events issues from the decision,
raising in one's favor all manner of unforeseen incidents
and meetings and material assistance,
which no man could have dreamed would have come his way.
Are you in earnest?
Seize this very minute.
Whatever you can do, or dream you can... begin it.
Boldness has genius, power and magic in it."

GOETHE

Meal Ideas

I like to eat fresh fruit as I prepare any meal. Sometimes the fruit and some vegetables or a big salad are all that I need. The main focus of at least one meal every day should be a large green salad. Then, if you'd like, add some steamed vegetables, a hearty soup, baked or steamed potatoes or yams, a cooked grain, or a legume dish.

HERE ARE SOME SIMPLE IDEAS (IN ADDITION TO THE MANY RECIPES IN THIS BOOK).

Mostly raw ideas

* FRUIT, our perfect food. If you eat enough this can be a good meal, maybe with some lettuce or celery. For example half a melon; or 2 apples, oranges, or mangoes; or 3 to 4 peaches; or bananas, etc.
* LARGE GREEN SALAD with a variety of lettuces, vegetables, nuts and seeds, avocado, olives, tomato, cucumber, sunflower and buckwheat sprouts, etc.
* ROMAINE LETTUCE (SLICED), AVOCADO (CUBED), MANGO (CUBED), COUPLE TABLESPOONS OF SAUERKRAUT — one of my favourite simple salads. Mangos are in season from April to June.
* VEGETABLES WRAPPED IN EZEKIEL 4:9 SPROUTED GRAIN WRAPS (a Food For Life product found in the freezer section of your health food store) — try cucumber, avocado, tomatoes, sprouts, sauerkraut, grated carrot, fresh herbs like basil, coriander, parsley, or chives, hummus or other spreads, almond butter.
* RAW VEGETABLES (carrots, pepper, celery, radishes, etc.) with dip
* Avocado wrapped in NORI SHEETS
* NUT OR SEED PÂTÉ with veggies, stuffed into a pepper, rolled in a lettuce, cabbage, or kale leaf
* BLENDED SOUP
* RAW ART ON A PLATE (see recipe) for a simple live meal
* WHEN I KNOW I WON'T BE HOME, I bring plenty of fresh fruit along with containers of a variety of washed and cut raw vegetables, soaked nuts or seeds, sprouted grain crackers or breads, dates or figs.

Some cooked ideas

Recipes for many of these ideas are in the recipe section. Accompany with raw vegetables or a salad.

* SANDWICHES WITH SPREADS: hummus, tofu salad, bean spread, tofu slices, nut butters, veggie patties, refried beans, cheese. Try a variety of breads and crackers: whole grain breads, pita pockets, buns, bagels, tortillas, rye crackers, rice cakes.
* STEAMED BABY NEW POTATOES, with yogourt and chives or blended avocado with lemon juice

* PASTA SALADS, RICE SALADS, TABBOULI, POTATO SALAD
* PIZZA: whole wheat pita or spelt/kamut crusts, tomato sauce, chopped veggies, grated cheese
* VEGETARIAN SUSHI
* GRAIN OR VEGETABLE PATTIES (or loaf) with potatoes, gravy, steamed vegetables
* CHILI. Try serving the chili on a bed of corn chips and shredded lettuce, and have fresh chopped tomatoes, onions, peppers, salsa, and guacamole on hand to garnish.
* PASTA WITH TOMATO OR OTHER SAUCE. Use whole grain pasta more often (brown rice, kamut, soba, etc.). I often add canned beans or lentils to a plain tomato sauce. Spoon fried onions, mushrooms, and/or green peppers over the sauce. Serve with a salad and/or steamed vegetables.
* STEWS
* CURRY and other Indian dishes
* MEAL IN A WRAP — a simple meal where everyone chooses their own stuffing
* VEGGIE BURGERS (patties made at home or bought ready-made). Try steaming pita pockets briefly, cutting them in half crosswise and stuffing them with burgers, tomatoes, sprouts, ketchup, mustard, relish, etc. Serve with OVEN-BAKED FRIES (potatoes cut in strips, tossed in a little olive oil and seasoned salt, and baked at 400F until golden).
* ORIENTAL OR THAI STIR-FRY over brown rice or other whole grain
* BAKED BEANS, big salad, or steamed vegetables
* LENTILS AND RICE
* TOFU TACOS with all the fixings
* GRILLED ASSORTED VEGETABLES, steamed grain, salad

Breakfast ideas

* FRESH FRUIT
* FRUIT SALAD
* SMOOTHIE, blender drink
* Fresh pressed FRUIT JUICE
* Fresh pressed GREEN JUICE
* LIVE PORRIDGE with optional nut milk
* SPROUTED GRAIN CEREAL
* ESSENE BREAD
* HOT CEREAL (oatmeal, cream of brown rice, cream of whole wheat, 7-grain, etc.) — serve with chopped fruit, raisins or berries, dried fruit, nuts and seeds, soy, nut or dairy milk, and a sweetener if desired
* WHOLE GRAIN CEREAL with rice, almond, or soy milk
* SPROUTED BREAD, toasted with nut butters and/or fruit-sweetened jam (try tahini and molasses on toast — an acquired taste maybe, but an excellent source of iron and calcium — many people love it, particularly my daughter)
* RICE CAKES with nut butters and/or jam or apple sauce or apple butter

* PANCAKES, WAFFLES, OR FRENCH TOAST with fresh fruit sauce
  (strawberries, blueberries, raspberries, etc. – fresh or thawed from frozen)
* Homemade MUFFINS
* SCRAMBLED TOFU on toast
* YOGOURT
* SOUP

Snack ideas

* FRUIT
* SMOOTHIE, blender drink
* NUTS AND SEEDS
* Figs, dates, apricots, currants, raisins, prunes, and other DRIED FRUIT
  (look for unsulphured)
* FRUIT LEATHER
* APPLE SAUCE
* RAW VEGETABLES with optional dip
* SPROUTED BREAD with coconut butter, hemp seed butter, pumpkin butter,
  or sesame butter
* CELERY STUFFED WITH NUT BUTTER
* SANDWICHES, pita pockets, or bagels
* SOUP
* FROZEN JUICE POPSICLE
* Organic POPCORN
* MUFFINS, COOKIES, OR LOAVES
* PUDDING
* YOGOURT
* WHOLE GRAIN CRACKERS with cheese
* RICE CAKES with nut butter, apple sauce, and a sprinkle of cinnamon
* RYE CRISPS with spreads
* CEREAL or porridge
* BAKED CORN CHIPS with salsa

"Whenever we cook for others,
we are making a statement to them.
If what we prepare and present
to our family and guests
is attractive, tasty, and health-supporting,
we are saying that we want them to be well and happy,
to feel nurtured and strengthened.
When we offer cuisine that is made of
whole and natural ingredients,
we are saying that we want them
to have all the energy they need
in order to make every aspect of their lives richer.
We are saying that we honor them."

JOHN ROBBINS, IN MAY ALL BE FED

Sample Menus

I eat about 70 to 90 per cent raw depending on the season, and my kids eat about 50 per cent raw. We are all lacto-vegetarians. Everyone's ideal diet varies according to many factors. However, it can help to get an idea how people balance a whole foods vegetarian diet. You will notice a difference between my kids and myself in the following typical days.

My typical day

In the morning I wait until I'm hungry to eat. Could be 8 am, could be 11 am (more often).

8 AM - 11 AM	Break fast with fresh fruit or fruit salad *Possibilities for later:* more fruit, green smoothie, wrap, soup, big salad, bowl of yogourt or kefir, raw vegetables, romaine hearts, raw nuts or sprouted bread or crackers
4 PM	Eat fresh fruit and or make a green juice while I prepare dinner
5 PM	Big salad or raw entrée, cooked or raw soup, and/or vegetarian meal

Jérémie's typical day

7 AM	Fruit salad or fresh fruit or smoothie, or whole grain cereal with rice milk, or sprouted grain bread with nut butter and jam
11 AM	*Lunch at school:* bean salad, or rice and bean salad, or pasta salad, or cheese sandwich with lettuce and tomato, or pizza on whole grain pita pockets, or soup or stew in a thermos, or burrito, or pita pocket with hummus and veggies; plus container of raw veggies, container of chopped fruit, apple, fruit leather, healthy muffin or square, or yogourt
3 PM	*After school snack:* fruit or rice cakes with nut butter and apple sauce, or smoothie, or yogourt
5 PM	*Dinner:* Big salad and/or soup, any whole grain or legume-based dish, steamed vegetables, or wraps
10 PM	*After hockey snack:* Turbo shake, or cereal with non-dairy milk, or soup, or bread with nut butter and jam

Jacqueline's typical day

7 AM   Fruit, fruit salad, smoothie, or nothing

11 AM   *At school:* big container of vegetables, or salad or a soup or a stew in a thermos; plus big container of prepared fruit (pineapple, melon, grapes, etc.), apple, fruit leather, healthy muffin or square

3 PM   (same as Jérémie)

5 PM   (same as Jérémie)

9 PM   *Evening or after volleyball:* fruit, or apple with peanut or almond butter, or smoothie, or cereal with rice, soy, or almond milk

3 weeks of quick dinners

The idea here is to show you how you can make wholesome meals for your family without spending hours in the kitchen. These should take you 30 minutes or less to prepare. However, you may have to think ahead and cook the grains or legumes earlier in the day. If there is a soup, you could make that in the morning or the night before. Soups consist of 10 minutes or so of chopping and then occasional stirring while it simmers. These suggestions could work Monday through Friday for 3 weeks. Notice how the grains and starches vary from day to day. Also, I generally try to emphasize raw foods every second dinner.

DECIDE WHAT YOU'RE GOING TO MAKE FOR THE NEXT SEVERAL DAYS, CHECK THE RECIPES AND ADD WHATEVER YOU NEED TO YOUR SHOPPING LIST.

WEEK 1

1. Greek Pasta Salad (p.153)
   Tip: cook noodles while you make the dressing and chop vegetables
2. Barley Mushroom Soup (p.126) with Cabbage Delight (p.162)
   Tip: make soup earlier in the day
3. Rice and Bean Salad (p.157) with a big green salad and any steamed vegetable
   Tip: cook rice and legumes earlier in the day
4. Meal in a Wrap (p.202) or Ezekiel 4:9 Wraps (p.219)
5. Hummus (p.121 or p.122) with veggies and Cashew Corn Chowder (p.128)
   Tip: make soup earlier in the day

WEEK 2

1. Baked Vegetables (p.231) and Baked Tofu Fingers (p.186)
   Tip: prepare vegetables and tofu earlier in the day and put in the oven 30 to 40 minutes before you're ready to eat
2. Live Miso Soup (p.144) with 4 F Salad (p.166) and any steamed vegetable in season
3. Quinoa and Tofu Salad Meal (p.156)
   Tip: bake the tofu and cook the quinoa earlier in the day

4. Cream of Green Soup (p.141) and Mashed Yams (p.233) and any salad or steamed vegetable
5. Lentils and Rice (p.199) and Kale Avocado Salad (p.167)
   Tip: cook the lentils and the rice earlier in the day

WEEK 3

1. Pasta with Beans and Greens (p.203) and spring mix with Balsamic Vinaigrette (p.171)
   Tip: cook pasta while you are chopping vegetables
2. Raw Art on a Plate (p.223) with White Bean Soup (p.138)
   Tip: make soup earlier in the day
3. Potato Salad (p.155) and Good Greens (p.232)
4. Soba Noodle and Greens Salad (p.158)
5. Guacamole Burritos (p.120) and Split Pea Soup (p.136)
   Tip: make the soup earlier in the day

Special occasions menus

RAW FOODS MEAL:
Veggie Pâté on yam slices (p.123)
Angel Hair with Marinara Sauce (p.218)
Marinated Portabello Mushrooms (p.233)
Green salad with Vinaigrette Dressing (p.176)
Apple-Fennel Salad with Lemon Zest and Thyme (p.160)
Orange-Nutmeg Dream Cake (p.255)

HOLIDAY FEAST MEAL (100% RAW):
Cream of Green Soup (p.141)
Guacamole with Sesame Flax Crackers (p.120, p.113)
Walnut Burgers with Ketchup à la Raw (p.227, p.179)
Carrot Beet Salad (p.163)
4 F Salad (now 5 F because it's Festive too!) (p.166)
Yam Pie with Cashew Cream (p.259, p.252)

WHOLE FOODS MEAL (50% RAW) FOR FALL-WINTER:
Lemony Tomato Tapenade on whole grain crackers (p.120)
Cream of Summer Squash (Zucchini) Soup (p.129)
Shepherd's Pie with Tamari Cream Gravy (p.206, p.183)
Steamed green beans or Good Greens (p.232)
Large salad with Greek Salad Dressing (p.173)
Banana ice cream with Caramel Sauce, berries, and chopped nuts (p.251)

Living Hummus with vegetables (p.121)
Gazpacho (p.143)
Pad Thai (p.221)
Mixed baby green salad with Balsamic Vinaigrette (p.171)
Baked Vegetables (seasonal – see recipe p.231)
Creamy Lemon Tarts (p.252)

HOLIDAY WHOLE FOODS MEAL (50% RAW):
Mushrooms stuffed with Nut Pâté (p.121)
Curried Squash-Apple Soup (p.130)
Eggplant Patties with Tamari Cream Gravy (p.195, p.181)
Root Fries or Mashed Potatoes (p.234)
Beets and Greens with Lemon-Basil Dressing (p.152)
Green salad with Dijon-Miso Dressing (p.172)
Living Date Squares with Cashew Cream (p.253, p.252)
Pecan-Fig Bars with Caramel Sauce (p.256, p.251)

BUFFET FOR KIDS AND FUSSY ADULTS:
Guacamole or Hummus and vegetables or crackers (p.120, p.121)
Pesto Soup or Cashew Corn Chowder (p.134, p.128)
Greek Pasta Salad (p.153)
Baked Potato Salad (p.150)
Baked Tofu Fingers (p.186)
Enchiladas (p.196)
Green salad with Vinaigrette Dressing (p.176)
Steamed vegetables (corn, green beans, carrots – see ideas on p.230)
Apple Crisp or Peach-Blueberry Crisp with Cashew Cream (p.238, p.244, p.252)

"If it doesn't taste good, it's not worth eating. If it doesn't bring you pleasure, it's not worth doing. Celebrate every one of your hungers. You will never be sorry." GENEEN ROTH

Menu plan – 75% raw vegan
"I eat with reverence and grace"

This menu plan is ideal for someone who wants to incorporate more raw into their diet. I have purposely left out dehydrated foods and other recipes that require much time to prepare and/or special equipment. It's also an excellent 5-day cleanse as it contains the least congesting food categories (fruit, vegetables, nuts, seeds, legumes, non-glutenous grains). However, if this is being adopted as a long-term diet, some raw dairy such as organic non-homogenized yogourt or kefir, raw cheeses, or goat feta could be added. Also, if there are digestive issues, more of the vegetables may have to be eaten steamed or blended.

NOTES FOR THE FOLLOWING DAYS
3 meals every day, to be eaten when hungry. I encourage people to wait until their body signals a comfortable hunger – back of the throat opens, stomach is receptive, emotions are clear, body is relaxed. So, for example, the first meal could be any-where between 7am and noon.

When you will be out of the house, prepare the food in the morning or the night before. Bring your first meal to be eaten when hungry. Make a smoothie or fruit salad and bring it with you in a glass jar or thermos. Other vegetables and fruit can be washed and placed in containers or jars.

Snack on fruit but make sure you eat that fruit at least 2 hours after a meal or 20 minutes before. I like to snack on fruit while I'm preparing lunch or dinner. A green smoothie also makes a nourishing and satisfying snack in the middle of the afternoon.

DAY 1
* MEAL 1: $1/2$ melon, or as much as need to feel satisfied, and later an apple or other fruit
* MEAL 2: Cabbage Delight (p.162)
  Later, snack on a rice cake with raw almond butter and sliced bananas.
* MEAL 3: Raw Art on a Plate (p.223), Lentil Soup (p.132)

DAY 2
* MEAL 1: Fresh pressed orange juice made from 3 or 4 oranges, and then enjoy the pulp afterwards too. Later, another seasonal fruit (maybe berries).
* MEAL 2: Large green salad with lettuce, sunflower sprouts and other sprouts, avocado, tomato, cucumber, olives, olive oil and lemon dressing. Could have a bowl of leftover Lentil Soup.
* MEAL 3: Greek Pasta Salad (p.153)

DAY 3
* MEAL 1: Fruit Salad Special (p.83)
* MEAL 2: Ezekiel 4:9 Wraps (p.219)
* MEAL 3: Angel Hair with Marinara Sauce (p.218), Good Greens (p.232)

DAY 4
* MEAL 1: 1 or 2 bananas and 1 mango, and later an apple or pear or other fruit
* MEAL 2: Raw vegetables and Hummus (p.121)
  A couple of hours later, snack on fruit or a green smoothie
* MEAL 3: Kale Avocado Salad (p.167), Baked Vegetables on quinoa (p.231)

DAY 5
* MEAL 1: Green smoothie (p.98)
* MEAL 2: 1 or 2 pears or apples or other fruit, 2 or 3 celery stalks (washed and cut up)
  or 1 romaine lettuce heart (washed), 1/2 avocado or 10 walnuts or almonds,
  fresh dates. Could bring some leftover baked vegetables too.
* MEAL 3: Quinoa and Tofu Salad Meal (p.156)

"Remember, every food purchase is a vote. We might be tempted, as individuals, to think that our small actions don't really matter, that one meal can't make a difference. But each meal, each bite of food, has a rich history as to how and where it grew or was raised, how it was harvested. Our purchases, our votes, will determine the way ahead. And thousands upon thousands of votes are needed in favor of the kind of farming practices that will restore health to our planet.

Our world can no longer afford the heedless consumption of the Western world that is now spreading its greedy tentacles around the globe. The price, most of which must be paid by our children, is too great. Only by acting together, by refusing to buy food that has been secretly laced with poisins and pain, can we make a stand against the corporate power that is circling our planet. So let us join hands. Let us speak out for the voiceless and the poor. Let us assert our right, as citizens of free democracies, to take back into our hands the production of our food. Let us, together, sow seeds for a better harvest—a harvest for hope." JANE GOODALL, IN HARVEST FOR HOPE

"The preparation of food also serves the soul
in a number of ways.
In a general sense, it gives us a valuable, ordinary opportunity
to meditate quietly, as we peel and cut vegetables, stir pots,
measure out proportions, and watch for boiling and roasting.
We can become absorbed in the sensual contemplation
of colors, textures, and tastes as, alchemists of the kitchen,
we mix and stir just the right proportions.
The colors and the smells can take us out of 'real' time,
which can be so deadening,
and lift us into another time and space altogether,
the time of myth created by cooking.
The kitchen is one of the most soulful rooms in a house,
often the center of family life."

THOMAS MOORE
IN THE RE-ENCHANTMENT OF EVERYDAY LIFE

Recipes

Recipes

"Using recipes as inspiration instead of rigid structures will allow your creativity to express itself and make cooking and eating more joyful experiences." ELEONORA MANZOLINI

Although I love to spend time preparing wholesome meals in my kitchen, like you, I lead a full life. The recipes that follow are a result of close to 17 years of experimenting in my kitchen. My intention is to give you recipes that are wholesome and simple. Often I start with recipes from favourite cookbooks and then modify with the purpose of making them with wholefood ingredients, simplifying, using less dishes and less time, and without compromising taste and healthiness.

WITH SINCERE APPRECIATION TO THE AUTHORS, HERE ARE SOME OF MY FAVOURITE COOKBOOKS/FOOD PREPARATION BOOKS AND NATURAL HEALTH BOOKS:

The American Vegetarian Cookbook From the Fit For Life Kitchen, by Marilyn Diamond
Ayurvedic Cooking for Westerners, by Amadea Morningstar
Conscious Eating, by Dr. Gabriel Cousens (L *)
Detox Your World, by Shazzie (L)
Eating for Beauty, by David Wolfe (L *)
Healing with Whole Foods, by Paul Pitchford (*)
The Hippocrates Diet and Health Program, by Ann Wigmore (L *)
Instant Raw Sensations, by Frederic Patenaude (L)
Living Cuisine, by Renee Loux Underkoffler (L)
May All Be Fed, by John Robbins and Jia Patton (*)
Moosewood Restaurant Cooks at Home, by The Moosewood Collective
The Pheylonian Cookbook, by Tahlia and Illah Chickalo
The Raw Gourmet, by Nomi Shannon   (L)
The Raw Truth, by Jeremy Saffron (L)
Salt Spring Island Cooking, by Rodney Polden and Pamela Thornley
Sunfood Cuisine, by Frederic Patenaude (L *)
The Sunfood Diet Success System, by David Wolfe (L *)
Vegetarian Times (a monthly publication) (*)
Any books by the Boutenko family (L)

* These books also have extensive sections on health and nutrition.
L These books focus on living foods.

Recipe Notes

In all recipes the following is implied unless otherwise stated: Use organic ingredients as much possible. Your body will thank you, the Earth will thank you.

tsp.   refers to teaspoon
Tbs.   refers to tablespoon
Milk   means to use soy, almond, rice, or dairy milk
Water   use the purest available: spring, distilled, reverse osmosis, filtered
Herbs   unless specified, measurements are for dried herbs but fresh are always
        preferable (usually 2 to 4 times more of a fresh herb)

Any unfamiliar ingredient may be listed in the glossary at the end of this cookbook.

When a recipe calls for an ingredient without measurements, assume that it is medium-sized. For example: "1 onion, chopped" can be understood as "1 medium-sized onion".

Symbols

(L)   after a recipe title means at least 95% of the ingredients in this recipe are living. I consider certain high quality yogourts and kefirs live because of the added life force and nutrients from the bacteria.

(G)   after a recipe title means that it contains no gluten—this is a protein found in many grains that creates digestive challenges and sensitivity or allergies in many people. Gluten-free also means wheat-free.

(S)   after a recipe means that it's made with sprouted grains which means that many of the nutrients, including the gluten are partially broken down so it's easier to digest.

(D)   after a recipe means that it's dairy free (most of the recipes in this book are), or there is a dairy-free option.

(T)+   after a recipe means that the preparation time is less than 20 minutes but it may require more soaking, cooking or dehydrating time while you can be doing something else!

(T)   after a recipe means that it can be prepared in less than 20 minutes.

If a recipe can not be prepared in less than 20 minutes, I have indicated the approximate time, which will not include soaking, simmering, baking or dehydrating time.

"The Seedling:

New life in any form is cherished by the forest friends:

the dawning of day, the emerging of plants, the unfolding of buds,

...and the birth of a child.

It is a time of joy, of hope, of renewed commitment to the Harmony credo.

New life is a gift and a treasure.

It must be carefully nurtured to allow and enable it

to develop to its fullest potential.

Lavish upon it the best of what you are, what you know, what you believe.

Show it the wonders of its world. Prepare it well for life.

A being strong in body, mind and spirit

is the greatest legacy we can leave behind."

MAIA HEISSLER

Breakfast

Buckwheat Grawnola

I love this cereal and make it in large batches —this is a great raw food breakfast for cold Canadian winters!

4 cups dry hulled buckwheat
   (will make 8 cups sprouted buckwheat)

1 cup raw almonds,
   soaked 4 hours, divided

1/3 cup sunflower seeds, soaked 4hours

1/3 cup pumpkin seeds, soaked 4 hours

1/4 cup flax seeds

1/4 cup sesame seeds

1 cup raisins or currants

SAUCE:

1 apple or pear

6 soft dates

1/3 cup soaked almonds (from above)

1 tsp vanilla or 1/2 vanilla bean
   (put the whole thing in skin and all)

1 tsp cinnamon

apple juice or water, enough to blend

honey, maple syrup or
   agave syrup to taste (optional)

pinch sea salt

1. Soak buckwheat for 12 hours, rinse thoroughly, and sprout for 2 to 3 days in a large colander. Rinse at least once a day until the tails are the same length as the grain. The water that runs off the sprouts will be slightly slimy—this is normal. Rinse well until the water is clear.

2. Drain, rinse and coarsely chop almonds (reserving 1/3 cup for sauce).

3. Drain and rinse sunflower and pumpkin seeds.

4. Grind flax and sesame seeds in a coffee grinder.

5. Blend sauce ingredients in a blender until smooth.

6. Place sprouted buckwheat, chopped almonds and all seeds in a large bowl. Pour sauce over top and mix until well coated.

7. Place mixture on teflex sheets on dehydrator trays in thin layers.

8. Dehydrate for 15 hours or so at 120F until completely dry.

9. Mix in raisins and store in an airtight container.

10. Serve with nut milk or rice milk.

Chai Kefir Ⓛ Ⓖ Ⓣ

I like to use Pinehedge Farm's Bio-Dynamic Kefir for this recipe. The milk is not homogenized and is sold in returnable glass jars. Any quality organic kefir or yogourt will do. Kefir is similar to yogourt but a different culture is used—it has an almost bubbly effect on the tongue and is sweeter than yogourt.

2 cups kefir or yogourt
1 small apple or pear, chopped
1 Tbs. grated coconut
1 banana sliced
1 to 2 Tbs. raisins or currants
1 Tbs. pumpkin seeds or sunflower seeds
1 Tbs. maple syrup or agave syrup
1/2 tsp. ground cinnamon
1/4 tsp. ground cardamom
pinch ground cloves
pinch allspice (optional)

1. Place all ingredients in a medium-sized bowl.
2. Stir to combine, being sure spices are equally distributed.

Serves 2 or 1 very hungry hockey player

French Toast Ⓓ Ⓣ

This is a respectable eggless version of a favourite breakfast food.

8 slices whole grain bread (try Ezekiel 4:9 sprouted bread from the health food store)
2 cups soy, rice or almond milk
3 Tbs. maple syrup
1 tsp. ground cinnamon
pinch of salt
small amount butter or coconut butter (for oiling cookie sheet)

1. Cut bread diagonally into triangles.
2. Combine milk, maple syrup, cinnamon, and salt with a whisk in a large shallow bowl.
3. Dip bread slices in batter until fully saturated.
4. Bake on a lightly oiled cookie sheet at 350F for 12 minutes. Flip with a spatula and bake for 10 minutes more until slices are browned and slightly crispy.
5. Serve with maple syrup and fresh or thawed berries.
Serves 2 to 4

Fruit Salad Special Ⓛ Ⓖ Ⓓ Ⓣ

What makes this fruit salad special is an abundance of juice. Fred Patenaude calls this fruit soup. Whatever you call it, it's a delicious way to break your fast in the morning. Because I like to delay my breakfast until I'm truly hungry, I serve this to my children in the morning before school and then put the rest in a wide-mouth jar for myself to take to work and enjoy when I'm ready.

SEASONAL FRUIT SUCH AS:

pears

bananas

grapes

kiwis

oranges

mandarins

berries (fresh or frozen)

pineapples

mangoes

apples

peaches

plums

nectarines, etc.

fresh pressed juice (orange or apple)

chopped dates, figs or raisins

1. Start off by cutting various fruit into bite-sized pieces and placing in a medium-sized serving bowl. Use what is available depending on the season, in any combination.

2. Then pour fresh pressed orange juice or apple juice over top, to cover. You could also use a store-bought fresh pressed juice or a high quality pasteurized juice like Wilde, Ceres, or many that can be found at the health food store, or combine various juices.

3. Sometimes I add chopped dates, figs, or raisins. The variations on this theme are endless.

4. A large bowl of this salad makes a light but satisfying breakfast.

Granola Ⓛ Ⓖ Ⓣ

This cereal is similar to many granolas found at the health food store. Making it yourself allows you to control the type and quality of ingredients.

4 cups rolled oats

2 cups spelt flakes

2 cups quick oats
  (or 2 more cups rolled oats)

1 cup unsweetened, shredded coconut

1/4 cup sesame seeds

2/3 cup sliced or chopped raw almonds

2/3 cup sunflower seeds or pumpkin seeds

1/4 cup spelt flour or whole wheat flour

1/2 cup sucanat

1 1/2 cups water

1 tsp. vanilla

1/4 cup cold-pressed coconut butter
  or expeller-pressed safflower oil

2/3 cup raisins, chopped dates, or
  apricots (or any other dried fruit)

1. Mix grains, nuts, and seeds in a large bowl.
2. Blend sucanat, water, vanilla, and coconut butter. Pour over dry ingredients and mix well.
3. Divide onto two large cookie sheets. Bake for 1 1/2 hours at 250F, stirring every 30 minutes, until dry.
4. Remove from oven, let cool, and put in a container, adding raisins or dates.

Makes 10 cups

Hearty Cereal Ⓛ Ⓖ Ⓣ

Use as a breakfast cereal, or as a snack, with any kind of milk (fresh nut milk is most whole-some) and sweetener if desired (we use sucanat). I leave a scoop in the container for easier serving. Use quinoa or buckwheat flakes and omit the oats for a gluten-free version.

4 cups whole grain cereal flakes
  (spelt, kamut, millet, buckwheat,
  quinoa, or corn flakes)

1 cup rolled oats

1/2 cup slivered almonds

1/4 cup sunflower seeds

2 Tbs. ground flax seeds

2 Tbs. sesame seeds

2 Tbs. hemp seeds

1/2 cup raisins, currants, or any other
  dried fruit (apples or apricots are great)

1/2 tsp. cinnamon

Anything else that you want to add in
  (coconut, chopped dates, other nuts)

1. In a large container or jar combine ingredients.
2. Mix well with your hands.

Makes 6 cups

Holiday Breakfast   Ⓖ Ⓓ Ⓣ

This has become a standard treat at Christmas and Easter Sunday. I buy Van's gluten-free waffles in the frozen section of my health food store.

Van's frozen waffles, toasted and
   kept warm in the oven

ICE CREAM:

Frozen bananas (peel ripe bananas,
   break into pieces and freeze in
   re-sealable bags or a plastic container)

TOPPING:

Frozen berries from our summer harvest
   (blueberries, raspberries, strawberries
   or a combination), thawed and
   mashed with a fork

Maple syrup

Dark organic chocolate crushed

Chopped nuts

Caramel Sauce - optional
   (see Raw Desserts)

---

1. *To make ice cream:* process bananas in a single- or twin-gear masticating juicer with the blank plate in place. You can also do this in a strong blender like BlendTech or Vitamix, starting with a small amount of bananas and gradually adding more as mixture gets smooth. Use a spatula to move bananas into blade and add a small amount of water as needed.

2. Serve ice cream on warm waffles and top with berries, syrup, chocolate, nuts and caramel sauce.

Live Rolled Grain Porridge Ⓛ Ⓢ Ⓓ Ⓣ

We ate this on a recent interior canoe/camping trip by putting the ingredients along with water together in a zip-lock bag at night. Up it went into the 'bear bag' with the rest of our food. The next morning we would enjoy it after yoga practice. We found it satisfying, easy to digest, and supportive of the energy demands of hiking and paddling. Sometimes I was lucky to have wild blueberries gathered from a hike.

1 cup large flake rolled oats, kamut, or spelt (or a combination of these)	1. Place in a bowl with enough water to cover by approximately 1/2 inch (1 cm.). Let soak overnight.
1/2 cup chopped or whole dried fruit (apricots, figs, dates, currants, prunes, goji berries, etc.)	2. The next morning, add a sprinkling of spices like cinnamon, cardamom, or nutmeg plus sweetener if desired (sucanat
1/4 cup raw nuts and/or seeds (almonds, sunflower seeds, pumpkin seeds, walnuts, pecans, etc.)	honey, maple sugar). Top with nut milk if desired.

Serves 1 to 2

Scrambled Tofu Ⓖ Ⓓ Ⓣ

My children enjoy this on toast, with ketchup of course! It makes a fast hearty breakfast, lunch, or dinner. Nutritional yeast, also known as Engevita yeast, is good tasting and adds B-vitamins and a cheesy flavour to dishes. As an option you can fry up some onions and peppers in the skillet and then add the tofu mixture. Delicious!

1 lb. firm tofu	1. In a medium-sized pot, mash all ingredients except water and cheese with a potato masher.
1 Tbs. nutritional yeast (optional)	
2 Tbs. olive oil or soft butter or coconut butter, or 1/2 and 1/2	2. Place pot on stove and cook over medium heat for 5 to 10 minutes. Add water and cook until desired consistency is reached, another 5 minutes or so.
1 Tbs. tamari	
1 heaping tsp. sea salt	3. Gently stir in optional cheese, allow to melt, and serve.
pepper to taste	
2 tsp. turmeric	4. Taste and adjust seasoning.
1/2 cup water	Serves 4
grated cheese (optional)	

Sunday Morning Crêpes

Light spelt flour has had some of the bran removed. It is ideal for occasional use such as in these crêpes or in pastries because it produces a lighter texture. This is the only recipe in this book with eggs.

2 organic eggs
1 cup milk (dairy, soy, or rice)
1/2 cup water
2 tsp. melted butter or olive oil
1 1/3 cups light spelt flour (or use whole wheat, spelt, or 1/2 whole grain with 1/2 all purpose flour)
1 tsp. honey
pinch of salt

PREPARATION TIME: 30 MINUTES

1. Combine all ingredients with a wire whisk, let sit for 5 minutes.
2. Pour a small amount of batter into a buttered frying pan, over medium heat, tilting the pan to spread batter as thinly as possible. Flip when golden and fry 1 more minute.
3. Serve rolled up with your choice of filling: fresh or frozen berries, apple sauce, yogourt or kefir, maple syrup, jam, honey, etc.

Serves 2 to 3

"Love is the most great law that ruleth this mighty and heavenly cycle, the unique power that bindeth together the diverse elements of this material world, the supreme magnetic force that directs the movement of the spheres in the celestial realms. Love revealeth with unfailing and limitless power the mysteries latent in the universe." ABDU'L-BAHA

"The Bird Track:

A Lakota proverb states that

'we will be known by the tracks that we leave behind'.

Tracks and associated signs and disturbances speak loudly

of the being who created them.

They can identify species, size, appetite, physical condition, and habits.

They tell whether the creature raced or ambled, if it fed, where it slept,

...what it crushed, even whether it cared about its surroundings.

In all we do, be it in our dealings with others,

in our attitude to the environment or in the work we do,

we leave signs as clear as bird tracks in freshly fallen snow."

MAIA HEISSLER

Juices and Beverages

Almond Chai ⓁⒼⒹⓉ⁺

A richly spiced creamy treat. Enjoy!

1 cup almonds, soaked 4 hours	1. Rinse soaked almonds and blend with water and all other ingredients at high speed until smooth.
4 cups fresh water	
1 1/2 Tbs. ginger	
2 tsp. cinnamon or 2 inches (5 cm.) cinnamon stick	2. Pour through a fine strainer, pressing with a spoon to remove all milk. Or use a nut milk bag available through www.carolinedupont.com or do a search for "nut milk bags" on the internet.
1/4 tsp. nutmeg	
1/2 tsp. cardamom	
1 tsp. allspice	
1/4 tsp. black pepper or 4 black pepper balls	3. Taste and adjust sweetness if desired.
pinch sea salt	4. Serve slightly warmed, chilled, or at room temperature.
1 tsp. vanilla extract	
1/4 cup soft dates (or soak 1/2 hour)	Serves 4
2 Tbs. raw honey	

"The experiment that would transform your world would operate upon the basic idea that you create your own reality according to the nature of your beliefs and that all existence was blessed and that evil did not exist in it." JANE ROBERTS AS SETH

Almond Milk Ⓛ Ⓖ Ⓓ Ⓣ⁺

This is my favourite milk alternative. It's delicious warm or cold. I also love to make this milk with 1/2 almonds and 1/2 sesame seeds. Try adding a few hazelnuts or brazil nuts. Some people add the almond fiber to cookies or use it in the shower as a body scrub!

1 cup raw almonds

4 cups water

1 Tbs. honey, agave syrup
  or maple syrup, to taste

1. Soak almonds overnight (or at least 4 hours) in enough water to cover by 1 inch (2 1/2 cm.).
2. Drain off water and rinse almonds several times.
3. Place almonds in a blender with 2 cups water and maple syrup.
4. Blend for 2 to 3 minutes.
5. Place a medium-sized fine strainer (lined with cheesecloth if desired) over a large bowl. Pour almond milk into strainer and allow to filter through. Or use a nut milk bag available through www.carolinedupont.com or do a search for "nut milk bags" on the internet.
6. Return almond fiber to blender and blend again with remaining 2 cups of water. Strain again.
7. Keep in fridge in a sealed glass container. Can be used over cereal or porridge, in baking, or in fruit smoothies. Delicious as is.

Makes approximately 5 cups

Blender Mineral Elixir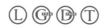

Here is how you can make green juice without a juicer.

2 Tbs. sesame seeds, or 1 Tbs. raw tahini	1. Blend all ingredients until smooth, approximately 2 minutes.
medium handful garden 'weeds' like dandelion and lambsquarters	2. Strain through medium strainer if desired. Feed the pulp to your dog!
small handful cilantro or parsley	3. This is a basic recipe and can be varied as you like.
big handful greens (spinach, kale, collards, lettuce)	
medium handful sprouts (pea, buckwheat, sunflower)	Serves 1 to 2
1/2 lemon, peel removed	
1 apple with peel, chopped	
1 inch (2 1/2 cm.) ginger	
1 large clove garlic, unpeeled	
1 Tbs. miso	
1/2 cucumber, chopped, leave peel on if it's organic	
1 1/2 cups pure water	
Optional: bit of celery, tomato, carrot	

Citrus Ambrosia ⓁⒼⒹⓉ

Here is a great way to enjoy a citrus beverage without wasting the goodness of the fiber and the white pith. Of course you can use any combination of citrus fruit – add a tangerine or use only oranges. Drink slowly and enjoy!

2 oranges
1 grapefruit
a few frozen berries

1. Peel fruit with a knife, leaving at least some of the white pith.
2. Cut into chunks, removing pits as you go along.
3. Place all fruit in a blender and blend for 1 to 2 minutes.
4. Strain through a medium strainer if desired to remove any coarse pieces.

Makes 2 servings

"...each human being has been created by God as a soul that will uniquely manifest some special attribute of the Infinite before resuming its Absolute Identity." PARAMAHANSA YOGANANDA

Fresh Juice Ideas Ⓛ Ⓖ Ⓓ Ⓣ

Fresh juices are one of the most powerful foods that you can add to your diet. Even if your health is not the best, you will benefit from all of the nutrients because these juices don't rely much on the digestive system and are absorbed at the level of the stomach and the duodenum (first part of the small intestine). I suggest one green juice every day, especially at the beginning of your health journey. Be sure to use organic produce!

GREEN JUICES – ANY FRESH JUICE MADE OF :
1. 50% celery and/or cucumber (less intense flavour than other greens, great alkalizers)
2. buckwheat sprouts and/or sunflower sprouts (packed with vitamins, minerals, and enzymes)
3. leafy greens (kale, spinach, Swiss chard, dandelion, lettuce, parsley, cabbage) (densely mineralized)
4. 1 apple, or 1 pear (to make it more palatable)
5. lemon, ginger, or garlic (optional)
6. small quantities of other vegetables such as carrots or beets (optional)

EXAMPLES OF GREEN JUICES (THESE WILL SERVE 1 TO 3 PEOPLE):
1. 3 celery stalks, handful spinach or kale, 3 carrots, small handful parsley, 1 apple, 1 lemon,
2. 1/2 cucumber, 2 celery stalks, 1 carrot, 5 leaves kale, handful wheat grass, handful sunflower sprouts, 1 lemon, 1 apple
3. 1 cucumber, 3 celery stalks, handful parsley, 5 large spinach leaves
4. large wedge cabbage, 1 large apple, 2 cups sunflower sprouts, 1 lemon, 1/2 beet, 2 celery stalks
5. 1 beet, 2 carrots, 6 kale leaves, 2 celery stalks, 1 apple

OTHER VEGETABLE JUICES:
1. Apple-celery: 3 apples, 3 celery stalks (no leaves)
3. Apple-beet-ginger-lemon: 3 apples, 1 beet, 1/2 inch (1 cm.) slice of ginger, 1 lemon
4. Carrot-apple: 4 carrots, 1 apple
5. Carrot-celery: 5 carrots, 2 stalks celery
6. Carrot-celery-apple-spinach: 3 carrots, 1 celery stalk, 1 apple, 1 cup spinach
7. Carrot-apple-beet: 4 carrots, 2 apples, 1 beet

Green Smoothies Ⓛ Ⓖ Ⓓ Ⓣ

A green smoothie is a fruit-based blender drink with added greens. It can be eaten as a meal and is the perfect way to get more greens and minerals into our diets in a delicious and satisfying way. They can be made in the morning and brought to work or school in a thermos or glass jar for an instant meal. There are limitless possibilities, but here are a few suggested combinations to start you off:

1 cup fresh orange juice,

1/2 to 1 cup fresh or frozen strawberries,

1 to 2 bananas, handful baby spinach

OR

1 apple, 1 pear

1 or 2 kale leaves, 1 stalk celery, water

OR

2 bananas, 1 cup kale, 4 dates,

1 cup apple juice

OR

3 peaches, 2 cups baby greens,

1 cup water or fresh apple juice

OR

1 mango, 1 cup pineapple,

big handful sunflower greens or

romaine lettuce, water

OR

1 apple or pear,

handful of sunflower greens,

1 celery stalk,

water, fresh apple or orange juice

1. Use added water or juice to achieve desired consistency. Green powders could also be added to these.
2. Blend for 1 to 2 minutes.

Jacqueline's Fruit 'Creamy'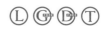

My 'smoothies' tend to get a little intense sometimes as I add more and more 'healthy' ingredients like spinach and green powders. This is my daughter's version of a truly delicious smoothie with no surprises!

2 bananas
1 cup fresh pressed orange juice
1 cup milk (almond, soy, rice) or any kind of juice (mango is nice)
1 cup fresh or frozen strawberries or raspberries
2 Tbs. maple syrup (optional – but not to Jacquie!)
6 ice cubes

1. Blend all ingredients on high for 1 minute.

Serves 2 very thirsty children and maybe a small cup for Mom too

"God Our Heavenly Father, You created the world to serve humanity's needs and to lead them to You. By our own fault we have lost the beautiful relationship which we once had with all your creation. Help us to see that by restoring our relationship with You we will also restore it with all Your creation. Give us the grace to see all animals as gifts from You and to treat them with respect for they are Your creation. We pray for all animals who are suffering as a result of our neglect. May the order You originally established be once again restored to the whole world..." Amen. SAINT FRANCIS OF ASSISI

Pink Ginger Lemonade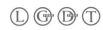

This lemonade has it all: it's tasty, excellent for the liver, can be a great sports drink, and it looks pretty.

2 lemons, peeled and chopped

1 pear, cored (or use an apple)

1/2 cup strawberries, raspberries, or blueberries

pinch Celtic sea salt (optional) – good if you want to use this as a sports drink

4 cups water

1 to 2 inch (2 1/2 to 5cm.) piece of ginger

2 to 3 Tbs. raw honey, maple syrup, agave syrup, or a combination

1. Blend well for 1 to 2 minutes.
2. Strain through a medium fine strainer.
3. Serve chilled.

Serves 4 to 6

Turbo Shake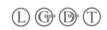

This shake was named by my son Jérémie, who loves to eat. When he comes home from hockey practice late at night, I make him one of these and leave it in the fridge in a big ceramic bowl-cup. Or I put it in a thermos and bring it in the car when I pick him up. The tahini and dates make it rich in calcium and iron. I keep frozen bananas in the freezer at all times for this and other blended treats or banana ice cream. When bananas are ripe, peel, break into pieces and place in a zip-lock bag or plastic container in the freezer.

2 small bananas, frozen or fresh

1 Tbs. raw sesame tahini

5 or 6 soft dates

2 to 4 Tbs. raw carob powder

1 Tbs. honey

1 tsp. vanilla

1 to 2 cups water (with some ice cubes if you are using fresh bananas)

1. Blend all ingredients for 1 to 2 minutes (depends on the power of your blender) starting with 1 cup of water and adding more water to reach desired consistency.

1 large or 2 small servings

"The Leaf:

The leaf is part of the tree and depends on it.

At the same time it performs its own function

toward the well-being of the whole.

It is a small but important part of a large picture.

The existence of the leaf is proof of the existence of the tree.

In the veins that bring it nourishment, every leaf bears the image of the

tree. Likewise every creature, somewhere, somehow,

bears the imprint of the Creator.

One should strive to recognize – and to honour –

the Creator in the creation."

MAIA HEISSLER

Breads, Muffins and Crackers

Baked Breads and Muffins:

Applesauce Muffins
Banana Bread
Blueberry-Orange Muffins
Breadmaker Recipe for Whole Grain Bread
Castle Bread
Essene Bread
Everything Bars
Orange-Oatmeal Muffins
Pear-Ginger Muffins

Raw Breads and Crackers:

Bagels
Living Buckwheat Crust
Sesame Flax Crackers
Sunny Flax Crackers
Sweet Potato Chips

Applesauce Muffins

1/2 cup milk (soy, almond, or dairy)

1 cup applesauce

3 Tbs. olive oil or butter

1/3 cup maple syrup or honey

1 Tbs. ground flax seed

2 cups whole wheat flour or spelt flour

1/2 tsp. salt

1 tsp. baking soda

1/2 tsp. cinnamon

1 to 2 Tbs. lemon zest

1 cup raisins or currants

1. Preheat oven to 375F. Lightly oil a 12-cup muffin pan, or two 12-cup mini-muffin pans with coconut oil.
2. Mix wet ingredients and flax seeds, set aside.
3. Combine dry ingredients and then add wet ingredients.
4. Add raisins. Fold together to combine.
5. Spoon the batter into the prepared muffin pan(s), filling each cup approximately 3/4 full. Bake until a toothpick inserted into the center of a muffin comes out clean (20 to 25 minutes for large muffins, 12 to 15 minutes for mini-muffins).
6. Let the muffins cool 5 minutes before removing from the pan.

Makes 12 large or 24 small muffins

Banana Bread

1/4 cup soy milk or almond milk

6 Tbs. olive oil, butter or coconut oil

6 Tbs. maple syrup

2 1/4 cups mashed ripe bananas
(approximately 5 medium bananas)

2 cups light spelt flour or
whole wheat flour

2 Tbs. roasted grain beverage powder
(Bambu, Caf-Lib, Inca) (optional)

1 tsp. baking soda

1 tsp. baking powder

1/2 tsp. salt

1 cup chopped walnuts or pecans

3/4 cup carob chips or
chocolate chips (optional)

1. Preheat oven to 350F.

2. Lightly oil an 8 inch x 8 inch cake pan or a loaf pan and dust with flour, shaking out excess.

3. Put the milk, oil, maple syrup, and bananas in a blender and blend until smooth.

4. In a large bowl, combine dry ingredients. Add the banana mixture and combine using as few strokes as possible. Fold in walnuts and optional chocolate chips or carob chips.

5. Pour into cake pan and smooth the top. Bake until a toothpick inserted into the center comes out clean (30 to 35 minutes).

Blueberry-Orange Muffins

1 1/2 cups freshly squeezed orange juice

1/3 cup olive oil or butter

1/3 cup pure maple syrup or honey

2 Tbs. tahini

Grated zest of 1 orange

2 cups whole grain flour
  (light spelt, kamut, or whole wheat)

1 cup rolled oats

1 tsp. baking powder

1 tsp. baking soda

1/2 tsp. sea salt

1 cup fresh or frozen blueberries, thawed

1. Preheat oven to 350F. Lightly oil a 12-cup muffin pan, or two 12-cup mini-muffin pans with coconut oil.
2. Put the orange juice, oil, syrup, tahini, and orange zest into a medium bowl and whisk until well-combined.
3. Mix the flour, oats, baking powder, baking soda, and salt together in a large bowl until well-combined. Add the orange juice mixture and combine, using as few strokes as possible so you do not overmix the batter. Fold in the blueberries.
4. Spoon the batter into the prepared muffin pan(s), filling each cup approximately 3/4 full. Bake until a toothpick inserted into the center of a muffin comes out clean (20 to 25 minutes for large muffins, 12 to 15 minutes for mini-muffins). Let the muffins cool 5 minutes before removing from the pan.

Makes 12 large or 24 mini-muffins

Breadmaker Recipe for Whole Grain Bread

I don't bake bread anymore, but below is the recipe for what was our favourite and many friends enjoyed as well. See if you can find Ezekiel flour at your Health Food Store. The grains are sprouted.

1 3/4 cups room temperature water

2 Tbs. olive oil

2 Tbs. honey

2 Tbs. molasses

1 1/2 tsp. salt

1 1/2 tsp. yeast (make sure your yeast is fresh – and keep it in the fridge)

4 cups flour –
Your choice of combinations:
I have often used light spelt flour. Otherwise I would use at least 1 cup of organic, unbleached, all-purpose flour for lightness, and the rest of the flour is a combination of spelt and whole wheat, sometimes with 1/2 cup of barley, kamut or rye flour.

1. Bake as you would any whole grain loaf in your breadmaker, following manufacturer's instructions.
2. I always make this bread on the Dough cycle. After the kneading and the first rising, I punch the dough down, knead it a little on a floured cutting board, put it in an oiled baking pan, let it rise a second time until doubled in size (40 minutes to 1 1/2 hour), and then bake it at 350F in the oven for 35 to 40 minutes.

Makes 1 large loaf

Castle Bread Ⓓ⁺ Ⓣ⁺

This is one of my neighbour Hrad's exotic bread creations. Since my interest in living foods is in the forefront these days, I no longer bake bread — my kids are more than happy to sample the various baked delights that he creates.

1 1/3 cup lukewarm water
2 Tbs. butter
2 Tbs. honey
1/2 Tbs. sucanat
3/4 tsp. sea salt
Cardamom seeds from 2 pods
1 tsp. fennel seeds
1 tsp. caraway seeds
2 cups hard white flour   (or light spelt flour)
7/8 cup whole wheat flour
1/8 cup rye flour
1 Tbs. buckwheat
2 Tbs. rolled oats
1 Tbs. rolled rye flakes
1 Tbs. rolled spelt flakes
2 1/4 tsp. yeast

1. Place in breadmaker on the 2 lb. setting in the order indicated. Or, alternatively, use the Dough cycle and after the first rising place the dough in an oiled bread pan and bake in the oven at 350F for 40 minutes.

Makes 1 large loaf

Essene Bread   Ⓢ Ⓓ Ⓣ⁺

Ideally all breads and crackers should be made from sprouted grains. Grains, which are not our natural food, become much easier to digest when they are sprouted because the sprouting process actually starts the digestion of grains for us. People who are sensitive to wheat or other glutenous grains find that they can often tolerate small amounts of sprouted grains. These loaves are also baked at low temperatures to preserve life-force.

2 cups kamut berries or wheat berries, soaked (becomes approximately 4 cups) (refer to instructions for soaking and sprouting at the end of the book)

FRUIT AND NUT VARIATION (MY FAVOURITE):

To the ground soaked berries add:

1 tsp. cinnamon

1/8 tsp. nutmeg

1/8 tsp. ground cloves

1/8 tsp. allspice

1/4 to 1/2 cup chopped dates and/or raisins

1/4 to 1/2 cup coarsely chopped nuts (for example: walnuts, pecans, or hazelnuts)

1. Soak berries for 12 hours.
2. Sprout berries 2 to 3 days, according to instructions, until sprouts are the same length as the berry.
3. Grind sprouts in a food processor or a Champion Juicer.
4. Knead for a few minutes, then shape into two flat 2 1/2 to 3 inch (6 to 8 cm.) high oval-shaped loaves.
5. Set on a cookie sheet.
6. Bake at 225F for 2 1/2 hours. Let cool.
7. Cut with a serrated knife.

Makes 2 small loaves

Everything Bars Ⓖ Ⓓ Ⓣ⁺

These bars have all nutrient categories covered—gluten-free grains, legumes, fruit, nuts and seeds, and vegetables so they are fully loaded. They are great anytime of the day and a satisfying snack or mini-meal on the go. The recipe can be doubled and frozen. Thank you Marjorie Hurt Jones, author of the Allergy Self-Help Cookbook for the inspiration for this recipe.

3/4 cup amaranth flour

3/4 cup buckwheat flour

1/2 cup quinoa flakes

1/2 cup chopped pecans or walnuts

1/4 cup sunflower seeds, or hemp seeds

1 tsp. baking soda

1 tsp. cinnamon

large pinch nutmeg, cloves, allspice

1/2 tsp. salt

3/4 cup chick peas

2/3 cup rice, soy or almond milk

1 banana

1/4 cup coconut oil

2 Tbs. tahini

1/3 cup honey, maple syrup
  or agave syrup

1 1/2 tsp. vanilla extract or
  3 inches vanilla bean, scraped

3/4 cup grated carrot or zucchini

1/2 cup currants, raisins or chopped dates

1. Preheat oven to 325F. Lightly oil an 8 inch by 10 inch baking pan.
2. In a large bowl mix together amaranth and buckwheat flour, quinoa flakes, nuts, seeds, baking soda, spices and salt.
3. In a blender or food processor combine chick peas, milk, banana, oil, tahini, sweetener and vanilla. Pour into the flour mixture and stir to combine. Add grated vegetables and dried fruit.
4. Pour batter (will be thick) into prepared pan and bake for 35 to 40 minutes, or until set.
5. Cool in the pan and cut into bars.

Makes 12 to 16 bars

Orange-Oatmeal Muffins

These muffins are the creation of my friend and colleague Ricki Heller. She's expert at creating delicious baked goods with whole foods ingredients. She also sells her baked goods at the Village Market in Thornhill on Saturday mornings and other places, and teaches vegetarian cooking, baking, and nutrition classes. You can find out about her and her services at www.rickiskitchen.com.

1 cup kamut flour or
  1 1/3 cups whole spelt flour

1 cup whole rolled oats

1 Tbs. baking powder

1 tsp. baking soda

1/3 cup chopped walnuts or other nuts

1/3 cup organic raisins

1/2 cup finely chopped dates
  (they should be soft)

1 organic seedless orange,
  washed, whole, and with skin

3 Tbs. olive oil or coconut oil

1/4 cup blackstrap molasses

2 Tbs. pure maple syrup

1/2 cup organic soy milk or other milk

2 Tbs. finely ground flax seeds

1. Preheat oven to 375F. Lightly grease 9 muffin cups for large muffins or 12 cups for smaller muffins (or line with paper liners).
2. In a large bowl, sift together flour, baking powder, and soda. Add raisins and walnuts, and toss to coat. Set aside.
3. Wash and dry the orange and cut into 8 sections. Process in a food processor until almost smooth (yes, the whole orange!). Next add the dates and process to a smooth puree. Add the oil, molasses, maple syrup, soy milk, and flax seeds and whir until well combined. (Tip: if you measure the oil first, then use the same cup for molasses and syrup, the last two won't stick!)
4. Pour the wet mixture over the dry ingredients in the bowl. Stir just until moistened. Spoon the batter into the muffin tins (large muffins will be quite full).
5. Bake in preheated oven for 20 to 25 minutes, until a tester comes out clean. Cool completely before storing. These are better the next day, as flavours meld. They also freeze beautifully.

Makes 9 to 12 muffins

Pear-Ginger Muffins

Another one of Ricki's wonderful muffins. See the previous recipe for more information on Ricki.

2 ripe pears, peeled, cored, and diced

2 tsp. ground cinnamon

1/4 cup finely chopped candied ginger
  or 2 tsp. freshly grated ginger root

1 cup light spelt flour

3/4 cup whole spelt flour

2 tsp. baking powder

3/4 tsp. baking soda

1/2 cup silken tofu

1/4 cup pure maple syrup

3/4 cup organic soy milk

1/4 cup extra-virgin olive oil

1/2 tsp. apple cider vinegar

1. Preheat oven to 375F. Lightly grease 9 muffin cups for large muffins or 12 cups for smaller muffins (or line with paper liners).

2. In a large bowl, combine the cinnamon, candied ginger (if using), flours, baking powder, and soda. Set aside.

3. In the bowl of a food processor, whir the tofu until smooth. Add the fresh ginger (if using), maple syrup, soy milk, oil, and vinegar and whir to blend. Pour the wet mixture over the dry ingredients and stir just to blend. Gently fold in the pears.

4. Spoon the batter into muffin tins (large muffins will be quite full). Bake in preheated oven 20 to 25 minutes, until a tester comes out clean. May be frozen.

Makes 9 to 12 muffins

Bagels ⓁⓈⒹ

My friend Mark first made these at a Batmitzvah that we were catering together. His were the most delicious that I have ever tasted. He baked them in the sun as well as the dehydrator. The following is my version of this lovely raw bread. These are great with a tahini/honey spread or almond butter. See the Sprouting section for more detailed instructions on how to sprout grains.

4 cups wheat kernels or kamut kernels, soaked 8 hours, drained, and sprouted for 36 hours

2 cups flax seed (can use a combination of gold and dark), soaked in 1 1/2 cups water for 4 hours

1 cup sesame seeds, soaked for 1 hour in 2/3 cup water

1/2 cup poppy seeds

1 Tbs. Celtic sea salt

1/3 cup olive oil

1/4 cup honey

PREPARATION TIME: 40 MINUTES

1. Run sprouted wheat and soaked flax seeds through a masticating juicer or process into a dough in a food processor. There will be some whole flax seeds remaining in the mixture.

2. Add remaining ingredients and mix thoroughly with hands.

3. Shape into round patties the width of a palm, approximately 5/8 inch (1 1/2 cm.) thick. Make a hole in the centre with your finger and place on dehydrator sheets.

4. Dehydrate at 140F for 3 hours and then at 110F for approximately 8 hours. Remove from sheets, flip and continue drying on trays until desired consistency is reached. I like them still slightly soft on the inside.

5. Store in a sealed container in the fridge. Makes approximately 24

THIS RECIPE, AND ALL OF THE RECIPES TO FOLLOW IN THIS SECTION ARE DRIED IN A DEHYDRATOR, WHICH DRIES FOOD WITHOUT 'COOKING' IT. BY DEFINITION, RAW BREADS AND CRACKERS SHOULD NOT BE HEATED ABOVE 118F, BUT OFTEN WE START WITH A HIGHER TEMPERATURE FOR THE FIRST FEW HOURS OR SO WHILE THERE IS A LOT OF MOISTURE IN THE DOUGH AND THEN TURN IT DOWN FOR THE REMAINING PERIOD. MANY DEHYDRATORS DO NOT HAVE TEMPERATURE CONTROLS AND DRY AT EXCESSIVE HEAT LEVELS. THE EXCALIBUR IS A GOOD BRAND WITH A THERMOSTAT AND MAY BE PURCHASED THROUGH YOUR LOCAL HEALTH FOOD STORES. IN CANADA YOU CAN ORDER ONE THROUGH WWW.HACRES.CA. FOR CRACKERS AND COOKIES YOU WILL NEED TEFLEX SHEETS TO LINE THE TRAYS. DEHYDRATION TIME VARIES ACCORDING TO THE MOISTURE OF THE DOUGH, AMBIENT TEMPERATURE AND HUMIDITY.

Living Buckwheat Crust Ⓛ Ⓖ Ⓓ Ⓢ

These crusts are a staple in our house. We use them as a base for raw pizza or hummus.
See the Sprouting section for more detailed instructions on how to sprout grains.

4 cups dry hulled buckwheat
  (will make 8 cups sprouted buckwheat)

4 large carrots, peeled

2 Tbs. dry oregano

1 cup flax seeds,
  soaked 4 hours in 1 cup water

1 Tbs. Celtic sea salt

1/3 cup cold pressed olive oil

4 Tbs. maple syrup, honey, or agave syrup

PREPARATION TIME: 40 MINUTES

1. Soak buckwheat for 12 hours and sprout for 2 to 3 days in a large colander, rinsing thoroughly at least once a day until the tails are the same length as the grain. The water that runs off the sprouts will be slightly slimy–this is normal. Rinse well until the water is clear.
2. Mix buckwheat, oregano, flax seeds, and salt in a bowl. Push everything through a blank screen juicer (for example: Champion or Green Power), alternating with the carrots. Add olive oil and sweetener. Mix batch thoroughly. Alternately, process all ingredients in batches in a food processor.
3. Using an ice cream scoop or an 1/8 cup measuring cup, place batter on dehydrator sheets. With a wet hand and circular movements, spread scoop until round crust is formed, approximately 1/4 inch (1/2 cm.) thick. Generally 6 fit on 1 sheet.
4. Dehydrate at least 15 hours, or until crusts are firm, crispy and completely dry, flipping halfway through if desired. Store in a sealed tight container.
5. Last at least 6 months if dehydrated thoroughly.

Makes 60 crusts

Sesame Flax Crackers

These delicious crackers are great with any dip or spread – or just on their own. I got the idea to add highly nutritious chia seed but simply omit them if you can't find them. I usually make them without garlic but suit yourself!

2 cups flax seeds
2 cups sesame seeds
1/2 cup chia seeds (optional)
2 Tbs. honey
1 to 2 cloves garlic (optional)
1 to 2 tsp. sun-dried sea salt

PREPARATION TIME: 40 MINUTES

1. Soak flax seeds and chia seeds in 3 cups fresh water for 4 hours.
2. Grind 1 cup sesame seeds in a coffee grinder or blender. Set aside.
3. In a food processor, mix soaked flax seeds (and optional garlic) in several batches, adding additional water if necessary to aid in blending. Continue processing to form a thick batter. The flax seeds will be broken but not necessarily smooth.
4. Transfer batter to a large bowl and add all ingredients, mixing thoroughly.
5. Spread the mixture in a thin layer on nonstick sheets on dehydrator trays using hands or moistened spatula for easier spreading.
6. Dehydrate at 110F for 12 to 20 hours until mostly dry. Cut into triangles, squares, or rectangles and return to dehydrator without nonstick sheets for 1 to 2 hours until completely dry and crispy.
7. Store in a plastic container in a cool dry place.

Makes a lot!

Sunny Flax Crackers

2 cups sunflower seeds,
  soaked 4 hours and rinsed

2 cups flax seeds,
  soaked 2 hours in 2 cups water

1 garlic clove (optional)

2 tsp. sea salt

1 heaping tsp. dried basil

1 heaping tsp. dried oregano

1 heaping tsp. dried thyme

PREPARATION TIME: 40 MINUTES

1. Process sunflower seeds, 1/2 of flax seeds, and optional garlic in a food processor or a masticating juicer until smooth. Transfer to bowl and add remaining ingredients.

2. Spread mixture 1/4 inch (1/2 cm.) thick on a dehydrator tray with a non-stick sheet. Wet hands to help in spreading.

3. Dehydrate at 110F for 10 to 12 hours until almost dry. Peel off nonstick sheets, score into desired cracker shapes, return to dehydrator (without nonstick sheets) and dehydrate until crispy (2 to 4 hours).

Makes a lot!

Sweet Potato Chips

3 cups peeled and shredded sweet potato

2 Tbs. lemon juice

1 cup sunflower seeds,
   soaked 4 hours and rinsed

1 cup almonds, soaked 4 hours and rinsed

1 cup flaxseeds, soaked in 1 cup water

1 cup chopped celery

1/4 cup red onion, chopped fine

1 clove garlic

3 Tbs. dried rosemary

1 tsp. thyme

1 Tbs. honey

1 to 2 tsp. sea salt

PREPARATION TIME: 40 MINUTES

1. Once the nuts and seeds have been soaked, start by shredding the sweet potato. A food processor works well but you can do it by hand.

2. Using the S-blade, process all ingredients in a food processor until smooth, adding water as necessary to help with blending. This can be done in batches.

3. Spread the mixture thinly on dehydrator nonstick sheets, using a spatula or wet hands for easy spreading.

4. Dehydrate at 110F for 10 to 12 hours until almost dry. Peel off nonstick sheets, score into desired shape, return to dehydrator (without nonstick sheets) and dehydrate until crispy (2 to 4 hours).

Makes a lot!

"The Snail:

The inward/outward spiral of the lowly snail is reminiscent
of powerful forces of wind and water.
The hard outer covering provides a retreat for protection and for recharging,
but the animal only moves forward when it emerges from its shell.
Similarly, the most powerful, violent storms are characterized
by fast-moving spirals of winds and clouds.
Yet at their centre there is calm.
Perhaps there is a correlation between
inner peace and outer strength."

MAIA HEISSLER

Dips and Spreads

Almond Mushroom Pâté

This lovely pâté is a delightful feast day appetizer on whole grain crackers. Idea: for quick crackers, I cut Ezekiel 4:9 wraps into squares and dry them on a cookie sheet in a warm oven (150F) until crisp.

1 cup blanched almonds

2 Tbs. finely chopped leeks
or mild onions

6 cups chopped mushrooms

3 Tbs. butter or olive oil

1 tsp. sea salt

1/2 tsp. thyme

pinch of pepper

1 tsp. honey

1 tsp. apple cider vinegar

1. Finely grind the almonds in a food processor or blender.
2. Sauté the leeks/onions and mushrooms in 2 Tbs. butter over medium heat until the liquid evaporates.
3. Add the spices, honey, and cider vinegar, and simmer until the mushrooms are almost completely dry.
4. Add this mixture to the almonds in the food processor, puree, blending in the remaining 1 Tbs. butter or oil. Taste and adjust seasonings.
5. Place in an attractive bowl, cover tightly, and chill at least a 1/2 hour.
6. Serve on whole grain crackers or toasted sprouted bread.

Makes 2 1/2 cups

Bean Dip   Ⓖ Ⓓ Ⓣ

1/2 cup onion (white or red), coarsely chopped	1. If using dried beans, see Reconstituting Dried Beans in the Soaking and Sprouting section at the end of the book.
1 Tbs. apple cider vinegar	2. In a food processor, combine onion, vinegar, cumin, chili powder, parsley, and optional peppers.
1 small clove garlic	
1/2 tsp. chili powder	
1/8 tsp. cumin	
1 to 2 chili peppers or hot sauce (optional)	3. Chop finely and gradually add drained and rinsed beans. Keep some liquid if needed for desired consistency. Taste and adjust seasonings.
small handful parsley or cilantro	
salt to taste	
one 14- or 15-ounce can white kidney beans, or black beans, or romano beans or one cup dried beans	4. Serve with baked corn chips, whole grain crackers, or raw crackers.

Makes 1 1/2 cups

Cottage Tofu   Ⓖ Ⓓ Ⓣ

Adapted from Marilyn Diamond's excellent cookbook American Vegetarian Cookbook this substitute for cottage cheese can be used whenever you would use dairy cottage cheese. It's nice as a spread and can be used in salads to replace feta.

1 lb. firm tofu	1. Place half the tofu and remaining ingredients in a blender or food processor and process to form a cream.
1 Tbs. olive oil	
1 Tbs. apple cider vinegar	2. Transfer to a bowl and set aside.
2 Tbs. fresh lemon juice	3. Mash the remaining tofu with a fork, then mix it into the blended portion and combine well.
2 Tbs. nutritional yeast (optional)	
2 Tbs. minced chives or green onions	
1 tsp. dried dill	4. Adjust seasonings to taste.
1/2 tsp. salt or salt-free seasoning	5. Refrigerate, tightly covered, until ready to use.

Makes 2 cups

Guacamole Ⓛ Ⓖ Ⓓ Ⓣ⁺

Avocados are satisfying and nutritious. This guacamole can be served with corn chips or rolled in a nori sheet with cucumbers, tomatoes, sprouts, and other grated veggies. Or try a raw burrito: spoon guacamole into individual romaine or leaf lettuce leaves, adding other veggies like sprouts, grated carrots, slivered cucumber, etc., roll lengthwise, and enjoy!

3 ripe avocados (approximately 2 cups when mashed)

2 cloves garlic, crushed

4 Tbs. lemon juice

1 tsp. sea salt or Herbamare

1 Tbs. flaked dulse (optional)

2 Tbs. minced chopped fresh sweet onion or green onion

for a chunkier version add finely chopped peppers (red, green, yellow), or broccoli, or chopped tomato

1. Mash avocado with garlic, lemon juice, salt, and dulse to desired consistency. I like to keep it a little chunky.
2. Add onion and optional vegetables.
3. Stir to combine and serve.

Makes approximately 2 cups

Lemony Tomato Tapenade Ⓛ Ⓖ Ⓓ Ⓣ⁺

Another one of Jacqueline's favourites. Serve it on crackers or toast.

1 cup sun-dried tomatoes, soaked for 1 to 2 hours

1/2 cup olive oil

1/2 to 1 tsp. salt

2 cloves garlic, crushed

1 1/2 tsp. grated lemon rind

1 1/2 Tbs. fresh lemon juice

1 tsp. chopped fresh thyme or 3/4 tsp. dried thyme

1 tsp agave syrup or other sweetener

1. Soak sun-dried tomatoes in warm water for 1 hour.
2. Drain and chop coarsely.
3. Process all ingredients in a food processor or blender until finely minced.
4. I make sprouted crackers for this by cutting Ezekiel 4:9 wraps into pieces and drying in a warm oven until crisp.

Makes 1 1/2 cups

Living Hummus   Ⓛ Ⓖ Ⓓ Ⓣ⁺

This recipe is inspired by raw food chef Jennifer Italiano — finally a raw hummus that tastes just as good as the cooked chick pea version!

3/4 cup almonds, soaked 4 hours	1. Drain and rinse nuts.
3/4 cup raw cashews, soaked 4 hours	2. Place all ingredients, except tahini,
2 Tbs. onion	in a blender and blend until smooth,
2 Tbs. garlic	scraping sides of processor to get mix-
1/2 cup fresh lemon juice (2 lemons)	ture into blades until it is very smooth.
2 Tbs. olive oil	Add water as needed to give desired
1 tsp. sea salt, to taste	consistency and to aid with blending.
pinch cumin	3. Add tahini and blend until thick.
1/2 to 1 cup water	4. Lasts up to 5 days in the fridge.
2 Tbs. raw tahini	

Makes 2 1/2 cups

Nut Pâté   Ⓛ Ⓖ Ⓓ Ⓣ⁺

Serve this pâté as a side dish to a raw meal, stuffed in a red pepper, or into mushrooms, or rolled into collard, lettuce, or cabbage leaves. Feel free to vary nuts and add different vegetables and herbs.

1/2 cup almonds	1. Soak nuts together for 4 hours, drain
1/2 cup combination nuts	and rinse.
(cashews, hazelnuts, walnuts,	2. Place nuts and remaining ingredients
sunflower seeds, more almonds)	in a food processor and process until
1/2 red pepper	smooth.
1 small tomato	3. You could also form this into a loaf
1 clove garlic	with tahini sauce over top (see salad
3 brown mushrooms	dressing section)
1 Tbs. lemon juice	
1 Tbs. sweet onion (optional)	Makes 1 1/2 cups
Celtic sea salt to taste	

Sherry's Heavenly Hummus

My friend Sherry and I, and our kids, were having a picnic one day and she brought this amazing hummus. I immediately asked her for the recipe. My heart sank when she told me that she skinned the chick peas in order to make it so smooth — all I could imagine was peeling all those chick peas one at a time. My days were already far too short! "No way", I thought, "this is where I draw the line". I stopped listening... But the more I tasted, the more open I became to the idea. Besides, she assured me that it was easy. And actually, it is. And it's well worth the little extra work.

2 cups skinned cooked chick peas (see explanation below), cooled or 2 cups canned chick peas (you cannot skin these ones – the hummus will not be quite as smooth unless you have a really powerful blender like BlendTech or Vita-Mix)

2 medium garlic cloves

1/4 cup fresh lemon juice

1/4 cup tahini

1/4 tsp. cumin

1/2 to 1 tsp. salt

reserved chick pea cooking liquid

TO SKIN CHICK PEAS :

1. Place 1 1/3 cups of dry chick peas in a medium- to large-sized pot and cover with water by 2 inches (5 cm.). Let soak overnight or at least 8 hours. This will make approximately 2 cups of cooked chick peas.
2. Drain. Rub 1 Tbs. of baking soda into chick peas and let sit 10 minutes.
3. Add water just to cover, and boil over medium-high heat for 5 minutes. Watch carefully, the mixture will foam easily – remove foam if needed.

4. Remove from heat and drain. Place pot in sink, cover chick peas with cold water and rub together with your hands. Skins will float to the top. Drain off water and skins and repeat until no more skins appear on the surface of the water.
5. Chick peas are now ready to cook. They will take approximately 20 minutes on low-medium heat. Let cool and use in recipe above.

TO MAKE HUMMUS:

1. Place garlic, lemon juice, and 1/2 cup of chick peas in blender. Blend until smooth.
2. Add the remaining chick peas, cumin, and salt (plus some of the reserved liquid to get desired consistency, if necessary). Blend until smooth and transfer to a bowl. Mix in tahini by hand.

Makes 2 cups

Tofu Salad Spread Ⓖ Ⓓ Ⓣ

Instead of egg salad. My daughter Jacqueline eats this by the forkful. If she leaves us some, we have it on rice or rye crackers or toasted sprouted or rice bread.

16 ounces firm tofu	1. Crumble the tofu finely into a medium bowl.
3 Tbs. minced celery	2. Add the remaining ingredients and mix well with a fork.
1 Tbs. minced green onion	3. Taste and adjust seasoning.
3/4 tsp. turmeric	
3/4 tsp. curry powder	
1/2 tsp. coriander	Makes approximately 3 cups
3 tsp. nutritional yeast	
1 tsp. salt or seasoned salt	
1/4 cup natural mayonnaise (I like Nasoya)	

Veggie Pâté Ⓛ Ⓖ Ⓓ Ⓣ⁺

A lovely raw pâté. Try serving it on slices of raw yam. Delicious! As an alternative, you can use 1/2 sunflower seeds and 1/2 pumpkin seeds.

1 cup sunflower seeds, soaked for at least 4 hours	1. Process sunflower seeds, carrot, cilantro or parsley, and garlic clove with the grinding attachment of a masticating juicer (for example: Champion or Green Power). Add remaining ingredients and mix well.
1 medium carrot	
1/2 cup cilantro or parsley	
1 clove garlic	
1 Tbs. lemon juice	2. Alternatively, blend all ingredients in a food processor or blender, except the miso and celery, until smooth, using a spatula to move mixture closer to blades. Mix in miso and celery by hand, and serve.
1 Tbs. mellow miso	
1 medium celery stalk, finely chopped	
	Makes approximately 1 1/2 cups

"The Rainbow:

This most colourful of Nature's light shows

symbolizes Hope and Promise for the Forest Friends.

It is a picture of Harmony and tells a story about diversity.

More than anything else, however,

the rainbow brings a message about simply taking delight

in beautiful things, things that often disappear mysteriously,

things that are short-lived.

Take time to marvel at the rosy dawn, the dance of the Northern lights,

the velvet patterns on the newly emerged moth.

To have witnessed a moment of beauty is to have enriched your soul forever."

MAIA HEISSLER

Soups

Cooked Soups:

Barley Mushroom Soup
Black Bean Soup
Cashew Corn Chowder
Cream of Summer Squash Soup
Curried Squash-Apple Soup
Kale and Navy Bean Soup
Lentil Soup
Miso Soup
Pesto Soup
Red Lentil and Barley Soup
Split Pea Soup
Vegetable Stock
White Bean Soup

Raw Soups:

Borscht Vitality Soup
Carrot Juice Soup
Carrot-Parsnip Soup
Cream of Green Soup
Garden Soup
Gazpacho
Live Miso Soup

Healing Soups:

Healing Soup #1: Orange Soup
Healing Soup #2: Green Soup
Healing Soup #3: Vegetable Soup

Barley Mushroom Soup

A satisfying and nourishing winter soup. Add a salad like Cabbage Delight and you have a meal.

1 cup barley, washed and soaked for 4 hours or overnight

1 Tbs. olive oil, butter, or sesame oil

10 button mushrooms, halved and sliced

1 1/2 cups leeks, halved, washed carefully to remove sand, and finely sliced (or use onion)

1 cup celery with leaves, halved and finely sliced

1 large carrot, grated

1/2 cup red lentils, rinsed

small handful hijiki or arame seaweed, crushed

1 to 2 tsp. Celtic sea salt

1 small bunch kale, large stems removed,washed and finely sliced (approximately 4 cups)

8 cups water or vegetable stock

2 Tbs. miso

1. Earlier in the day or the night before, soak barley in fresh water at least 4 hours. Drain and rinse.

2. In a large soup pot, heat oil and gently sauté mushrooms, leeks, celery, and carrot until tender, adding water as necessary to prevent sticking.

3. Add barley, lentils, seaweed, salt, kale, and water or vegetable stock. Bring to a boil and then turn down heat, simmering for 30 minutes until barley is tender.

4. Remove approximately 1/2 cup of liquid from soup and mix in miso until dissolved. Return to soup, taste, and adjust seasoning. Avoid boiling soup once miso has been added.

Serves 6

FOR COOKED SOUPS, I GENERALLY USE WATER TO START; OR IF I REMEMBER, I KEEP THE COOKING WATER FROM MILD VEGETABLES AND USE THAT. FOR COMPANY, I MIGHT MAKE A VEGETABLE STOCK (YOU CAN FIND A RECIPE IN THIS SECTION). IF THE SOUP IS LACKING DEPTH ONCE COOKED, I MIGHT ADD A TEASPOON OR TWO OF CONCENTRATED VEGETABLE BOUILLON (HERBAMARE AND GAYLORD HAUSER ARE GOOD BRANDS). ALL SOUP RECIPES CAN BE DOUBLED.

Black Bean Soup   Ⓖ Ⓓ Ⓣ⁺

This is a delicious soup with an exotic flavour. Try serving it with fresh chopped parsley, cilantro and/or chives. And maybe a dollop of yogourt or kefir? Very hearty and satisfying.

2 cups dry black beans, soaked and cooked (2 cups dry = 5 cups cooked, see instructions to the right) – or 2 to 3 cans black beans (enough for 5 cups)

10 cups water or vegetable stock

1 large onion, finely chopped

2 cloves garlic, minced

2 carrots finely grated

2 stalks celery, finely chopped

1/2 cup fresh parsley

3 Tbs. molasses

3 Tbs. tamari

2 Tbs. olive oil, coconut butter, or ghee

2 bouillon cubes or 2 tsp. vegetable broth powder

2 tsp. cumin

2 tsp. coriander

1 heaping tsp. Celtic sea salt

1/2 tsp. ground cloves

cayenne pepper or hot sauce, to taste – anything to add fire

1. Soak beans overnight (or at least 8 hours) in water to cover by 4 inches (10 cm.).

2. Discard soaking water and rinse several times.

3. Bring beans and 10 cups water or vegetable stock to a boil, turn down heat and cook 1 to 2 hours until beans are tender enough to be mashed easily on the roof of your mouth with your tongue. Add extra water if necessary so that the soup contains the full 10 cups water (allow for evaporation). Beans should be covered by 2 to 3 inches (6 to 7 cm.).

4. In a large skillet, heat oil or butter on medium and gently sauté onion, garlic, carrots, celery, and parsley until very tender. Then add sautéed mixture to beans along with the remaining ingredients.

5. Cook on medium for 15 to 20 minutes to blend flavours. Adjust seasonings and serve hot. Garnish as desired with fresh herbs, or yogourt.

Serves 6 to 8

Cashew Corn Chowder

Children love this soup. The secret to its sweet creaminess is blending part of the cooked soup with raw cashews.

6 cups water

1 1/2 cups chopped leeks or onions

2 celery stalks with leaves

3 cups diced potatoes

4 cups corn (fresh off the cob or frozen)

1 cup fresh parsley, minced, or
  2 Tbs. dried parsley

1 tsp. dill weed

1/2 tsp. tarragon

1/2 cup raw cashews

1 tsp. sea salt

1. In a large soup pot bring water to a boil.
2. Add the leeks or onions, celery and the potatoes, return to a boil, and then turn down heat to simmer until vegetables are soft, about 15 minutes.
3. Add the corn, parsley, and herbs. Continue cooking for 10 minutes.
4. Remove approximately 3 cups of this mixture and blend with cashews for approximately 1 minute until very smooth. Make sure there are no cashew pieces left.
5. Add cashew-corn milk to remaining soup. Season with salt and pepper if desired.

Serves 6

Cream of Summer Squash Soup

Ever wonder what to do with those huge zucchinis, also known as summer squash, that seem to double in size overnight? This is a wonderful simple soup that everyone enjoys.

1 Tbs. olive oil or butter

1 1/2 cups leeks or onions

8 cups coarsely chopped summer
squash (zucchini)

2 potatoes, washed and chopped

small handful parsley, coarsely chopped

water or vegetable broth
(see instructions)

salt and pepper, to taste

1. Gently sauté leeks or onions in oil or butter until soft and lightly browned.

2. Add summer squash, potatoes, parsley, and enough water or broth to reach the level just below the vegetables. Be careful, summer squash is very watery and if you add too much water your soup will be too thin.

3. Simmer soup for approximately 20 minutes, until squash is tender.

4. Blend soup in batches until very smooth, adding salt and pepper to taste.

Serves 6

Curried Squash-Apple Soup

A lovely fall soup with interesting flavours.

1 large butternut squash, peeled and chopped coarsely, approximately 4 cups (or substitute pumpkin or other squash)

1 leek, washed and finely chopped

2 cloves garlic, minced

1 Tbs. ginger, peeled and minced

1 medium apple, cored and chopped (leave skin on if you have a very powerful blender)

water, enough to cover soup ingredients, approximately 4 cups

3/4 tsp. ground cinnamon or 3/4 inch (2 cm.) cinnamon stick

2 tsp. ground coriander (or use 2 tsp. whole seeds)

1 tsp. ground cumin seeds (or use 1 tsp. whole seeds)

1 Tbs. raw honey

2 Tbs. coconut oil

1 tsp. turmeric

Celtic sea salt, to taste

tamari or nama shoyu 1 to 2 Tbs. (optional)

PREPARATION TIME: 30 MINUTES

1. In a large soup pot bring 3 cups water to boil and add squash, leek, garlic, ginger, and apple. Add more water, enough to just cover vegetables.
2. Gently simmer for approximately 10 minutes, until squash can be easily pierced with a fork.
3. Grind cinnamon, coriander, and cumin if using whole spices. (A coffee grinder works well.)
4. Add remaining ingredients to soup, including spices.
5. Process the soup in batches in a blender until smooth.
6. Taste and adjust seasoning.

Makes 4 to 6 servings

Kale and Navy Bean Soup   Ⓖ Ⓓ Ⓣ⁺

A one- dish meal that warms the soul. You can serve it with a sprinkling of raw organic parmesan or Swiss cheese.

1 cup navy beans, soaked overnight
6 cups water
2 tsp. olive oil
1 cup chopped onion or leek
1 large stalk celery with some leaves
1 large carrot, grated
1 small bunch kale (or collards) – thick stems removed and chopped
2 tsp. thyme
1 Tbs. vegetable broth powder
1 Tbs. tamari
1 to 2 tsp. sea salt
pepper to taste

1. Drain and rinse navy beans. Place in a medium-sized pot with 6 cups water. Bring to a boil, lower heat and simmer until tender, about 1 1/2 hours.

2. In a large soup pot, heat oil over medium heat and gently fry onion or leek, celery and carrot, until vegetables soften. Add kale and fry a few more minutes.

3. Add cooked beans to vegetable mixture, along with cooking water, thyme, vegetable broth, tamari, salt and pepper.

4. Simmer 15 minutes or so until kale is soft, taste and adjust seasoning.

Serves 4 to 6

Lentil Soup Ⓖ Ⓓ Ⓣ⁺

One of the best ways to get people excited about legumes is through delicious, hearty soups. Legumes can tend to leave a dry sensation in the mouth – soups make them more juicy and they absorb the flavours of the broth that they are immersed in. In exchange, they add a richness to the broth itself and a fullness to the finished soup.

6 to 7 cups water or vegetable stock

1 cup lentils (green or brown),
  picked over and rinsed

1 medium leek or onion, finely chopped

1 medium carrot, finely chopped

1 celery stalk, finely chopped

4 garlic cloves, pressed or minced

one 14-ounce can pureed tomatoes
  or tomato sauce

1/2 tsp. dried thyme,
  or 1 tsp. fresh thyme

2 tsp. balsamic vinegar

2 tsp. honey

1 heaping tsp. Celtic sea salt

fresh black pepper, to taste

1. Bring water to boil in a large soup pot and add lentils, leek or onion, carrot, celery, and garlic.
2. Gently simmer for 40 minutes until lentils are very tender
3. Add tomatoes and thyme and simmer for approximately another 15 minutes, adding extra water if necessary.
4. Stir in vinegar, honey, salt, and pepper. Serve hot.

Serves 4 to 6

Miso Soup Ⓖ Ⓓ Ⓣ

This is a basic miso soup recipe. These soups are light and delicate. Miso is a salty fermented grain product used in Japan as a base for soups. Miso can be found at your local health food store. Being fermented, it is rich in live enzymes. A few details to pay attention to: vegetables should be cut small, the soup should not be boiled once miso has been added, and always add some sort of fresh vegetable such as green onions just before serving.

3 cups water (as pure as possible)

1 to 3 Tbs. seaweed, soaked for
20 minutes in warm water, then rinsed
(hijiki, arame, wakame work fine –
start with a small amount and increase
to your liking)

1 cup thinly sliced, small diced, or
shredded vegetables (onions, carrots,
daikon radish, cabbage, winter squash,
yam, celery, etc.)

2 Tbs. barley miso or brown rice miso

Green onions, thinly sliced, for garnish
[or any other fresh and raw food such
as grated carrot, chopped parsley,
fresh ginger, or grated daikon
(Chinese radish)]

1. Bring water and seaweed to a boil
over medium heat. Reduce heat to low,
cover, and simmer for approximately
5 minutes.

2. Add vegetables and simmer covered,
over low-medium heat for 3 to 4 minutes,
until just tender.

3. Remove 1/2 cup of hot broth into a
cup, add miso, and stir until dissolved.

4. Stir miso mixture into the soup,
garnish with green onions, and serve
hot. Do not boil the soup after the miso
has been added as this destroys the
beneficial enzymes.

Serves 2 to 3

Pesto Soup   Ⓖ Ⓓ Ⓣ⁺

This recipe comes from my Mom's kitchen. We all love it! For a dairy free version, omit the parmesan and sprinkle the soup with Pine Nut Parmesan (see recipe).

10 cups water

1 1/2 cups each: diced carrots, diced
  potatoes, diced white of leek or onion

2 tsp. Celtic sea salt

1 1/2 cups green beans,
  in 1 inch (2 cm) sections

2 cups canned kidney beans or
  romano beans (drained and rinsed)
  or 1 cup dried kidney beans

1/2 cup broken whole-grain spaghettini
  or vermicelli (rice pasta works well)

1 slice stale bread, crumbled

1/3 tsp. pepper (optional)

PESTO:

4 cloves garlic, pressed or minced

6-ounce can tomato paste

1/4 cup fresh basil or
  1 1/2 Tbs. dried basil

1/2 cup parmesan cheese (optional,
  L'Ancêtre, a company in Québec
  has a lovely raw version)

3 Tbs. olive oil

1. If using dried beans, see Reconstituting Dried Beans in the Soaking and Sprouting section at the end of the book.

2. Gently simmer water, vegetables, and salt in a large soup pot for 30 minutes. Then add both types of beans, pasta, bread, and pepper. Simmer 15 more minutes.

3. Meanwhile whisk together pesto ingredients in a bowl. Add to soup just before serving.

Serves 6 to 8

Red Lentil and Barley Soup

A satisfying, nourishing soup with flavourful mild Indian spices.

1/2 cup barley, soaked a few hours	1. In a large pot heat oil and gently fry onions, celery, ginger and garlic for a few minutes. Add spices and fry another few minutes.
1 Tbs. olive oil	
1 cup onion or leek, chopped	
1 stalk celery, chopped	2. Add remaining ingredients and cook for 30 minutes or so, until lentils are tender. Remove bay leaves before serving.
1 tsp. ginger, grated	
1 tsp. garlic, minced	
1/2 tsp. ground coriander	Serves 4 to 6
1/2 tsp. ground cumin	
1/2 tsp. turmeric	
pinch cayenne pepper	
1 cup carrots, halved and sliced	
1 tomato chopped (or a small can of diced tomatoes)	
handful fresh parsley, chopped	
a few collard or kale leaves (stems removed and chopped) or a handful baby spinach, chopped	
2 bay leaves	
1 tsp. sea salt, to taste	
4 cups water	
1/2 cup red lentils	

Split Pea Soup Ⓖ Ⓓ Ⓣ⁺

A vegetarian version of a French Canadian classic. The yam gives it a satisfying sweetness. To decrease gassiness caused by legumes and pulses eat them with a simple salad and/or steamed vegetables.

8 cups water

1 leek or onion, diced

2 celery stalks with leaves, diced

2 carrots, diced

1 large yam or sweet potato, chopped

2 cups yellow or green split peas,
  picked over and rinsed

1 1/2 tsp. oregano

2 bay leaves

1 tsp. salt (or to taste)

pepper, to taste

1. Place water, leek or onion, celery, and peas in a large pot and simmer for 30 minutes over low-medium heat.
2. Add yam, carrots, and seasonings. Simmer for another 30 minutes, until peas and vegetables are tender.
3. Blend in batches and return to pot. Add salt and pepper to taste. Serve hot.

Serves 6

Vegetable Stock Ⓖ Ⓓ Ⓣ⁺

You can use not-so-fresh vegetables to make this stock. Enjoy this stock on its own sipped from a mug, as a rich base for soups, or as the cooking liquid for grains. It can be stored in the refrigerator in a glass jar for 3 to 4 days. It also freezes well.

10 cups water

2 medium onions, chopped

2 ribs celery with leaves, chopped

2 medium carrots unpeeled, chopped

2 medium baking potatoes unpeeled,
  chopped

1 head garlic unpeeled,
  cut in half horizontally (optional)

4 sprigs parsley, chopped

2 bay leaves

1/2 tsp. sea salt

1/2 tsp. black peppercorns

1. In a large pot, combine all the ingredients and bring to a boil over high heat. Reduce the heat to low and simmer, partially covered, for approximately 3 hours.
2. Pour the stock and vegetables into a strainer set over a large bowl. Discard or compost the solids remaining in the strainer.

Makes 10 cups

White Bean Soup ⒼⒹⓉ⁺

Serve this hearty soup with a big salad for a wholesome meal.

4 cups water or vegetable stock

1 cup leeks or onions,
   chopped medium fine

1 rib celery, finely chopped

1 large garlic clove, minced or pressed

2 Tbs. olive oil

1 medium red bell pepper, chopped

1 bay leaf

1/2 tsp. ground fennel

1 large potato, cubed

handful baby spinach, coarsely chopped

1 Tbs. Tamari

1 Tbs. fresh lemon juice

2 cups canned white kidney beans,
   drained and rinsed (16-ounce can),
   or 1 cup dried

Ground black pepper to taste (optional)

Sea salt, to taste

Chopped fresh parsley

1. If using dried beans, see Reconstituting Dried Beans in the Soaking and Sprouting section at the end of the book.

2. In a soup pot, gently fry the leeks or onions and garlic in the oil until softened.

3. Add water or vegetable stock, pepper, bay leaf, fennel, and potato and continue to cook for approximately 10 minutes, stirring regularly.

4. Add spinach to the pot along with the Tamari, lemon juice, and water. Cover and simmer for 10 more minutes until potatoes are tender.

5. Stir in the beans and gently reheat. Add black pepper and salt to taste.

6. Garnish with parsley and serve.

Serves 4

Borscht Vitality Soup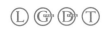

This fresh soup is 100 per cent raw. Exceptionally nutritious and satisfying.

1 medium-sized beet, coarsely chopped

1/2 inch (1 cm.) slice ginger

1 clove garlic, chopped

1 carrot, coarsely chopped

1 stalk celery, coarsely chopped

1 avocado, coarsely chopped

1/2 cucumber,
   peeled and coarsely chopped

juice of 1 orange

1 tsp. sea salt

1 tsp. dill

1 to 2 cups water

1/4 head cabbage, grated

1 small carrot, grated

fresh chopped parsley

clover or alfalfa sprouts, for garnish

1/4 cup chopped walnuts or pecans,
   for garnish

1. In a blender or food processor, process beet, ginger, garlic, first carrot, celery, avocado, cucumber, orange juice, Bragg's (or salt), and dill until smooth, gradually adding water until desired soupy consistency is achieved.
2. Pour mixture into a large bowl and add grated cabbage, carrot, and parsley. Adjust seasoning with salt.
3. Serve at room temperature, or in hot weather refrigerate until chilled (at least 2 hours).
4. Serve in individual bowls garnished with sprouts and chopped walnuts.

Serves 3 to 4

MOST RAW SOUPS REQUIRE A BLENDER OR FOOD PROCESSOR. THE BLENDING OFTEN HEATS UP THESE SOUPS SLIGHTLY, WHICH MAKES THEM MORE INVITING IN THE WINTER TIME. ALSO, USE ROOM TEMPERATURE INGREDIENTS AND SERVE IN BOWLS THAT HAVE BEEN WARMED IN THE OVEN.

Carrot Juice Soup Ⓛ Ⓖ Ⓓ Ⓣ

The live version. Thanks Fred Patenaude.

1 cup celery juice (from 3 to 4 celery stalks)	1. Juice celery and carrots, reserving 1 cup of the carrot pulp.
2 cups carrot juice (from approximately 8 carrots)	2. Blend juice with avocado and herb (dill or cilantro).
1 cup carrot pulp	3. Place this mixture in a bowl and add remaining ingredients.
1/2 avocado	
small handful of dill or cilantro	
2 medium tomatoes, diced	Serves 2 to 3
1/2 cup diced cucumber	
1 green onion, finely sliced	
1/2 avocado, diced	
pinch salt, to taste	

Carrot-Parsnip Soup Ⓛ Ⓖ Ⓓ Ⓣ

This simple recipe was passed on by a student after a raw foods seminar. I happened to have just bought some lovely parsnips from my friend and master bio-dynamic farmer Joe Born so I went straight home and tried it. I was surprised and pleased!

2 parsnips	1. Blend all ingredients in a blender until smooth.
1 carrot	
1 avocado	
2 Tbs. lemon juice	Makes 1 large or 2 small servings
pinch of salt, to taste	
water, enough for a smooth consistency	

Cream of Green Soup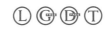

A lovely green soup inspired by Roxanne's Live Food Restaurant in California.

4 cups baby or young spinach (loosely packed)
1/2 avocado
2 Tbs. celery
1 Tbs. nama shoyu or tamari
1 Tbs. + 1 tsp. lemon juice
2 tsp. green onion or chives
1 tsp. garlic
1 1/2 tsp. fresh tarragon (or 1/2 tsp. dried tarragon)
1 sprig thyme (or a big pinch dried thyme)
1 1/2 cups water
pinch cayenne
salt and pepper, to taste
olive oil, to taste

1. Blend all ingredients until smooth.
2. Strain through a medium strainer, if desired.
3. Garnish with a splash of olive oil, and/or finely chopped green onion or red pepper.

Serves 2 to 4

Garden Soup Ⓛ Ⓖ Ⓓ Ⓣ

This delicious soup is adapted from Annie and David Jubb's Lifefood Recipe Book.

1 cucumber, chopped

1 red pepper, chopped

2 stalks celery, chopped

1 medium tomato

1 apple, cored and chopped

1/4 cup lemon juice

1 inch (2 1/2 cm.) ginger root,
   peeled and finely chopped

1 whole cloves garlic, chopped

1/2 cup chopped red or sweet onion

1 to 2 bushy stems cilantro or parsley

3 Tbs. fresh ground sesame seeds
   (use a coffee grinder) –
   or use 2 Tbs. tahini

2 Tbs. unpasteurized miso

2 Tbs. olive oil, or hemp seed oil,
   or flax seed oil

pinch cayenne (optional)

2 1/2 cups water

1. Blend all ingredients on high for 2 to 3 minutes until smooth. You may have to do it in two batches depending on your blender.

2. Will keep for 36 hours. Great in a thermos for lunch the next day.

Serves 2 to 4

Gazpacho ⓁⒼⒹⓉ

May be the mother of all raw soups?

6 cups ripe fresh summer tomatoes	
1 large cucumber, peeled	
1/2 green pepper	
1 red pepper	
2 green onions	
1 clove garlic, chopped	
1 Tbs. lemon juice	
salt or salt-free seasoning, to taste	
1/4 cup chopped fresh cilantro	

1. Set aside 1/3 of the cucumber and 1/3 of the tomatoes. Chop these into small cubes.
2. Set aside a slice of green pepper, and 1/3 of the red pepper. Cube finely.
3. Puree the rest of the ingredients (except for cilantro) in a blender on medium-high for approximately 1 minute until smooth.
4. Add reserved vegetables and chopped cilantro. Chill.

Serves 4

"To grow into the fullness of the Divine is the true law of human life and to shape his earthly existence into its image is the meaning of his evolution."

V.T. NEELAKANTAN, MYSTICISM UNLOCKED (OF KRIYA BABAJI)

Live Miso Soup Ⓛ Ⓖ Ⓓ Ⓣ

We first tasted this delicious soup at The Other Side Café in Newmarket. It has since become a staple in our home. Nori, dulse, and arame are seaweeds you can find at your local health food store. Miso is a salty fermented grain product used in Japan as a base for soups—being fermented, it's rich in live enzymes as well as beneficial bacteria. You can vary the type of miso used (barley, rice, white, dark, etc.).

3 cups pure water

2 to 3 dried shitake mushrooms,

1/2 sheet nori, cut with scissors into strips (fold nori and cut on angle with kitchen scissors to form short strips)

small handful dulse, cut into pieces with scissors

2 Tbs. dried arame or hijiki seaweed, crushed

2 to 3 Tbs. unpasteurized miso (in the refrigerator section of your health food store)

1/2 green onion, finely chopped

sesame seeds

2 to 3 tsp. tahini

1. Warm water in a medium-sized pot over very low heat until it is just hot to the touch.
2. Turn heat off, add mushrooms and let sit, covered, for approximately 10 minutes, until mushrooms are tender. Remove mushrooms with a slotted spoon and chop.
3. Return mushrooms as well as nori, dulse and arame or hijiki to the pot and let sit another 5 minutes or so, covered.
4. Remove 1/2 cup of broth from the pot into a cup and mix with miso until dissolved. Return to pot. Taste and add more miso if necessary.
5. Serve in individual bowls, topping with green onions and sprinkling generously with sesame seeds.
6. Let each person stir 1 tsp. of tahini into their bowl if desired.
7. If reheating this soup, watch carefully and only let it get warm to the touch.

Serves 2 or 3

Healing Soup #1: Orange Soup

4 cups orange vegetables, coarsely
chopped, any combination
(yam, carrot, squash, small rutabaga)

2 medium potatoes (skin on), cubed

2 celery stalks with leaves,
chopped medium fine

1 leek, chopped medium fine (optional)

Celtic sea salt, to taste

pure water

1. Place prepared vegetables in a pot
and add enough pure water to just
cover the vegetables.

2. Gently simmer for 20 to 40 minutes,
until vegetables are tender.

3. Blend soup until smooth in a blender
or with a hand blender, adding more
water if necessary

Serves 4 to 6

THIS SOUP AND THE FOLLOWING 2 SOUPS ARE HEALING IN
THAT THEY ARE ENTIRELY MADE OF VEGETABLES, WITH NO SPICES, NO ADDED FAT, AND
VERY LITTLE OR NO SALT. (PEOPLE WITH CANCER ARE BEST TO AVOID SALT COMPLETE-
LY). THEY ARE PERFECT FOR PEOPLE COMING OFF A FAST, WHO ARE SICK, OR WHO HAVE
DIGESTIVE INFLAMMATION AND ARE UNABLE TO TOLERATE RAW VEGETABLES FOR THE
TIME-BEING. SOMETIMES, INSTEAD OF SALT I BLEND IN 1 OR 2 TABLESPOONS OF MELLOW
MISO AT THE END OF COOKING.

Healing Soup #2: Green Soup

4 to 6 cups packed green vegetables, coarsely chopped, any combination (spinach, kale, swiss chard, broccoli, collards, handful parsley)

2 medium potatoes (skin on), cubed

2 celery stalks with leaves, chopped medium fine

1 leek, chopped medium fine (optional)

Celtic sea salt, to taste

pure water

1. Place prepared vegetables in a pot and add enough pure water to just cover the vegetables.
2. Gently simmer for 20 to 40 minutes, until vegetables are tender.
3. Blend soup until smooth in a blender or with a hand blender, adding more water if necessary.

Serves 4 to 6

"I suggest that since we are inseparable parts of the whole, we can enter into a holistic state of being, become the whole, and tap into the creative powers of the universe to instantaneously heal anyone anywhere." BARBARA ANN BRENNAN

Healing Soup #3: Vegetable Soup

Use any vegetables in this nourishing soup. As an option, you could add broken rice pasta at the end of cooking to please little ones.

2 celery stalks, chopped medium fine

1 leek, chopped medium fine

2 carrots, halved and sliced

1 1/2 cups cabbage, sliced fine

1 yam, cubed (or 1 cup squash)

2 potatoes, cubed

1 1/2 cups chopped spinach or kale

1 cup Jerusalem artichoke, cubed
(optional) – NOT French artichokes
("Jerusalem artichoke" is a root that
tastes somewhat like a potato –
it's easiest to find in the fall)

1 cup cauliflower, coarsely
chopped (optional)

Scarborough Fair seasoning:
handful parsley (chopped fine),
1 tsp. sage,
1 tsp. rosemary (crushed),
1 tsp. thyme – or any herbs that you like.

For a tomato base add a little tomato
sauce or crushed tomatoes –
I use frozen summer harvest Roma
tomatoes which I blend before adding
to the soup.

Celtic sea salt, to taste

pure water

1. Place prepared vegetables and herbs into a large pot and add enough water to cover by 4 inches (10 cm.).

2. Gently simmer for 20 to 40 minutes, until vegetables are tender.

Serves 8

"The Twisted Root:

the root spends its life probing deep into the earth

in order to anchor and nourish the tree that will touch the heavens.

This is its sole – and very significant – function.

The root does not allow itself to be stopped by obstacles.

It simply changes its course, it branches out, it finds a way to continue.

Its every twist and turn is a story of an obstacle overcome.

Sometimes, in places that abound in shattered stones,

the root will even absorb a piece of rock.

The root is shaped by its surroundings, not stopped by them.

It is a story of determination and persistence."

MAIE HEISSLER

Salads

Salads with a little help from the stove:

Baked Potato Salad
Bean Salad
Beets and Greens with Lemon-Basil Dressing
Greek Pasta Salad
Lentil Salad
Potato Salad
Quinoa and Tofu Salad Meal
Rice and Bean Salad with Cashews
Soba Noodle and Greens Salad
Wild Rice and Broccoli (or Fiddlehead) Salad

Raw salads:

Apple Fennel Salad
Arame-Yam Salad
Cabbage (or Broccoli) Delight
Carrot-Beet Salad
Chinese Cabbage Salad
Dandelion-Pear Salad
Earth Bowl
4F Salad (Favourite, Fast, Flavourful and Filling)
Kale Avocado Salad

Baked Potato Salad Ⓖ Ⓓ Ⓣ⁺

The longer this salad cooks, the more the flavour intensifies and wraps itself around the tender potato chunks. You can serve it warm but I prefer it at room temperature. Great in lunches the next day.

1 cup water
2 Tbs. tamari
2 cloves minced garlic
1/2 cup finely chopped red onion
2 Tbs. apple cider vinegar
3 Tbs. olive oil
2 tsp. dried tarragon, crushed
1 kg (2 lbs.) small new red or white potatoes (unpeeled), quartered

1. Preheat oven to 350F.
2. Combine all dressing ingredients (all but the potatoes) in a shallow 3-quart casserole.
3. Quarter the potatoes and add to casserole. Toss to coat.
4. Bake uncovered until potatoes are fork tender and golden (approximately 1 1/2 hours), stirring occasionally.
5. Serve at room temperature.

Makes 4 cups

"You are part of Divinity. Feel it, realize it, and all ties will drop away and you will be free. The attainment of this freedom through self-knowledge will bring you to the realization of your oneness with Divinity." V.T. NEELAKANTAN, MYSTICISM UNLOCKED (OF KRIYA BABAJI)

Bean Salad Ⓖ Ⓓ Ⓣ⁺

A classic hearty salad and a great addition to any vegetarian buffet. Canned beans are conven-
ient and work fine in this recipe. However preparing them from dried beans is more nutritious.

BEANS AND VEGETABLES:

2 cups cooked kidney beans
(from 1 cup dry)

2 cups cooked pinto beans
(from 1 cup dry)

2 cups cooked chick peas
(from 1 cup dry)

1 lb. green beans, in 1 1/4 inch (3 cm.)
sections, lightly steamed

1/2 cup finely chopped red onion
or sweet onion

1 small red pepper, diced

2 stalks celery, diced

DRESSING:

1/4 cup olive oil

1/4 cup apple cider vinegar

3 Tbs. sucanat

salt, to taste

1. If using dried beans, see
Reconstituting Dried Beans in the
Soaking and Sprouting section at the
end of the book.
2. Because beans take varying amounts
of time to cook, each type of bean will
be soaked and cooked separately. Soak
beans overnight and drain and rinse
well. Place beans in individual pots and
cover with 1 inch (2 1/2 cm) of water
and simmer over low heat until tender,
45 minutes to an hour and a half. Beans
should be very tender (no crunch left).
3. In a saucepan gently warm oil,
vinegar, and sucanat until dissolved.
4. Add to drained beans as well as all
remaining ingredients, and toss until
coated.
5. Let sit overnight in the fridge.
Season to taste.

Serves 12 to 15

Beets and Greens with Lemon-Basil Dressing ⓖ ⓓ ⓣ⁺

Rich in bone-strengthening silicon, beets sedate the spirit, improve circulation, purify the blood, strengthen the heart, and benefit the liver. This salad is particularly delicious in the late summer/early fall when beets are first being harvested with their greens. At other times of the year I have replaced the beet greens with spinach or Swiss chard.

12 small or 6 medium beets (with greens)

3 Tbs. freshly squeezed lemon juice
  (4 if not using raspberry wine vinegar)

1/4 cup olive oil

1 Tbs. raspberry wine vinegar (optional)

1/2 tsp. sea salt

1/8 tsp. freshly ground black pepper

1/2 cup chopped fresh basil

1/4 to 1/2 cup crumbled feta (optional)

1. Cut greens from beets. Scrub beets well. Wash beet greens in a sink full of cold water – cut leaves into 3/4 inch (2 cm.) strips and stems into 1/2 inch (1 cm.) strips.

2. Put 1 1/4 inches (3 cm.) of water in a large saucepan with a steamer basket, add beets, cover with the lid and bring to a boil. Lower heat and steam until tender, 15 to 30 minutes depending on size of beets. Remove from steamer basket with a spoon and let cool.

3. Add the beet stems and leaves to the pot and steam for 3 to 5 minutes, until tender.

4. Mix all dressing ingredients, except basil and feta, in a large serving bowl.

5. Peel beets by running them under cold water, then halve and slice them. Transfer to serving bowl.

6. Transfer beet greens and beet stems to bowl and toss.

7. Just before serving, add the fresh basil and the optional feta. Serve warm, chilled, or at room temperature.

Serves 4 to 6

Greek Pasta Salad Ⓖ Ⓓ Ⓣ

A meal in a bowl that takes less than a 1/2 hour to prepare. Make the dressing in the bottom of the salad bowl and simply start adding the rest of the ingredients. I have found this to be a kid pleaser. Use rice pasta for a gluten free alternative.

1/4 kg (1/2 lb.) pasta
  (shells, spirals or rotini)
  (rice, kamut, or wheat)

DRESSING:

3 Tbs. olive oil

2 to 3 Tbs. lemon juice

1/2 to 1 tsp. salt or Herbamare

1 large or 2 small cloves garlic

1 tsp. dried dill (or 1 Tbs. fresh dill)

1 tsp. dried oregano
  (or 1 Tbs. fresh oregano)

VEGETABLES:

1 pepper (red, yellow, orange,
  or green, or a mixture)

1/2 English cucumber, diced
  (peeling is optional)

2 tomatoes, diced

1 celery stalk, sliced

2 green onions, finely sliced

1 can chick peas (2 cups) or
  1 cup dried chick peas

1 cup crumbled feta or firm tofu

handful Greek olives

1. If using dried chick peas, see Reconstituting Dried Beans in the Appendix section at the end of the book.
2. Bring a large pot of water to a boil, add pasta and cook until tender but firm, drain, rinse under cold water, drain again.
3. Meanwhile, prepare dressing with oil, lemon juice, garlic, salt, and herbs in the bottom of a large salad bowl.
4. Add prepared vegetables, chick peas, feta or tofu, olives, and pasta.
5. Toss to coat. Taste and adjust seasoning.

Serves 4 as a meal

Lentil Salad Ⓖ Ⓓ Ⓣ⁺

Easy and flavourful. Bring leftovers to work the next day or send it to school with your children.

LENTILS:

1 cup brown lentils

4 cups water

2 bay leaves

1 tsp. fresh thyme or 1/2 tsp. dried thyme

2 cloves garlic, peeled

DRESSING:

3 Tbs. olive oil

2 Tbs. red wine or balsamic vinegar
   (you could also replace completely
   or partially with lemon juice)

1/2 tsp. ground fennel

3/4 tsp. Dijon mustard

salt and ground pepper, to taste

VEGETABLES:

1/2 cup diced celery

1/2 cup diced red or yellow pepper

1/4 cup minced red onion

1/2 cup chopped fresh parsley

1/3 cup crumbled raw sheep feta
   or goat feta (optional)

1. Rinse the lentils. In a medium-sized saucepan, bring the lentils, water, bay leaves, thyme, and garlic to a boil. Reduce the heat and simmer for approximately 20 minutes, until tender, stirring occasionally.

2. Combine the dressing ingredients in a large bowl. Add the celery, pepper, onion, and parsley.

3. Drain the lentils and discard the bay leaves. Remove the garlic, mash it, and add to dressing. When lentils are cool, toss with the vegetables and dressing and add the crumbled feta.

4. Adjust seasonings. Serve at room temperature.

Serves 4

Potato Salad ⒼⒹⓉ⁺

A healthy enjoyable version of a classic. There are two alternatives for the dressing: originally I made this using a store-bought tofu-based mayonnaise, but lately we've been enjoying it with a homemade avocado dressing.

1 1/2 pounds small potatoes, preferably new (unpeeled and scrubbed)

DRESSING:

1/2 cup natural mayonnaise
  (or 1 large avocado blended with
  2 Tbs. lemon juice and 2 Tbs. water)

1 Tbs. Dijon mustard

1/4 cup chopped fresh parsley,
  or 1 Tbs. dried parsley

1/4 cup chopped fresh dill,
  or 1 to 2 tsp. dried dill

1 to 2 tsp. fine sea salt
  or Herbamare, to taste

VEGETABLES:

1 large carrot, quartered length-wise
  and finely chopped

2 ribs celery with leaves, finely chopped

1 cup peas (fresh or frozen)

2 Tbs. finely chopped onion

paprika

1. Cut potatoes into bite-sized pieces, place in a steamer basket and steam until fork tender (15 to 20 minutes). Set aside to cool.

2. Put the mayonnaise (or avocado mixture), mustard, parsley, dill, salt, and pepper into a small bowl and stir to combine.

3. Add the carrot, celery, peas, and onion.

4. Add cooled potatoes and toss to coat.

5. Serve at room temperature.

6. Sprinkle with paprika.

Serves 3 or 4 as a meal,
more as a side dish

Quinoa and Tofu Salad Meal   Ⓖ Ⓓ Ⓣ⁺

This is a prototype for any kind of salad meal and a good way to start introducing more raw foods to your meals. All you need is some sort of grain and/or a legume, some raw vegetables, and any dressing. It's quick and allows for creativity — no two salad meals are ever the same! To simplify, I start by making the dressing in the bottom of a large salad bowl and then add the rest of the ingredients, choosing them by looking for variety in colour and flavour, and chopping vegetables in various shapes and sizes.

1/3 to 1/2 cup Asian Dressing
   (see recipe section Dressings)

TOFU CUBES:

1/2 lb. firm tofu

1 Tbs. tamari

1 tsp. olive oil

QUINOA:

3/4 cup quinoa

1 1/2 cups water

1/2 tsp. salt

VEGETABLES:

4 cups sliced romaine lettuce or
   red leaf lettuce or baby salad mix

1 cup sunflower sprouts

1/2 cup red cabbage, sliced very thin

2 green onions, sliced

1/2 English cucumber, cubed

1/2 red pepper or yellow pepper, sliced

other vegetables (carrot slices,
   radish slices, snow peas) (optional)

2 Tbs. sesame seeds

1. Chop tofu into cubes (slightly larger than dice). Place in a shallow pan and toss with tamari and olive oil. Bake at 350F for 20 to 25 minutes until lightly browned. Set aside to cool.

2. Meanwhile, rinse quinoa and place in a medium-sized saucepan, adding water and salt. Bring to a boil on high, cover, and reduce heat to low for 15 to 20 minutes, until all liquid is absorbed and quinoa is tender. Set aside and let cool.

3. Place prepared vegetables in a large salad bowl and add cooled tofu and quinoa. Top with dressing and sprinkle with sesame seeds. Serve immediately.

Serves 3 to 4 as a meal

Rice and Bean Salad with Cashews

As a nice alternative, try this salad with cooked quinoa and black beans. Serve with a green salad for a complete meal. My son Jérémie really enjoys this one. Good in school lunches.

DRESSING:

2 Tbs. lemon juice or red wine vinegar

1 Tbs. tamari

3 Tbs. olive oil

1 clove garlic, minced

1/4 tsp. oregano

SALAD:

2 cups cooked brown rice, cold
   (from 3/4 cup cooked in
   1 1/2 cups water)

1 cup cooked and cooled red kidney
   beans or chick peas,
   from 1/2 cup dried (or use canned)

3 green onions

2 celery stalks, finely chopped

1/4 cup fresh parsley

1/2 cup raw cashews, coarsely chopped

1. If using dried beans, see Reconstituting Dried Beans in the Soaking and Sprouting section at the end of the book.

2. Mix together lemon juice, tamari, olive oil, garlic, and oregano in a medium-sized salad bowl. Let stand 30 minutes if possible.

3. Mix together all other ingredients and pour dressing over top.

4. Toss to combine. Best eaten at room temperature.

Serves 4 to 6

Soba Noodle and Greens Salad

This is another flavourful version of a meal-in-a-bowl with both raw and cooked ingredients. It's quick to prepare and satisfying to eat.

10 ounces buckwheat soba noodles
  (or any other thin noodles like udon)
  – found at health food stores

DRESSING:

1 tsp. toasted sesame oil (optional)

2 Tbs. cold pressed sesame oil

1 medium clove garlic, finely minced

1/2 tsp. ground cinnamon

1/2 tsp. ground cumin

2 tsp. minced fresh ginger

2 Tbs. rice vinegar (or use lemon juice)

2 Tbs. tamari or nama shoyu

1 Tbs. maple syrup or agave syrup
  or honey

VEGETABLES:

2 to 3 stalks celery, sliced on the
  diagonal into 1/2 inch (1 cm.) strips

3 to 4 cups sliced bok choy, thinly sliced

2 to 3 green onions, sliced lengthwise
  in half and then sliced

1 carrot, grated

1/4 cup cashews, chopped

1. Cook the noodles in boiling salted water until tender. Drain and rinse under cold water. Drain thoroughly and separate noodles gently with your hands.
2. Mix oils, garlic, spices, vinegar, tamari, sweetener, and salt in the bottom of a large bowl.
3. Transfer the noodles, the prepared vegetables, and the cashews to this large bowl. Mix gently.
4. Serve at room temperature.

Serves 2 as a meal, 6 as a side dish

Wild Rice and Broccoli (or Fiddlehead) Salad ⒼⒹⓉ⁺

Wild rice is not a true rice. The grains are the seeds of a North American aquatic grass. Wild rice is never refined. It has a distinctive nutty flavour and as it cooks, the grains pop open and curl attractively. If you could find some wild leek instead of onions, and even some fiddleheads instead of the broccoli, you will have a truly wild salad! Wild leek and fiddleheads are found at local markets for a limited time in the spring time. Thank you Evelyne, www.heartycatering.com.

3/4 cups wild rice, washed and
    soaked 4 to 12 hours

2 1/4 cups fresh water

3 cups broccoli florets (or fiddleheads)

1 large carrot coarsely grated

1 Tbs. fresh lemon rind

1/3 cup red onion, minced
    (or use chives or wild leeks)

1/2 cup fresh parsley, minced

1/2 cup walnuts, chopped

DRESSING:

3 Tbs. extra virgin olive oil

2 Tbs. lemon juice

1 tsp. honey or maple syrup

1 tsp. Dijon mustard

Sea salt and pepper to taste

1. Cook wild rice in water for 40 minutes, or until all grains pop open and curl. Set aside to cool.

2. Cook broccoli or fiddleheads until tender-crisp. Set aside and let cool.

3. Combine dressing ingredients in the bottom of a large attractive bowl.

4. Add rice, broccoli, and remaining ingredients. Toss gently to combine.

5. Taste and adjust seasoning.

Serves 4

Apple-Fennel Salad with Lemon Zest and Thyme

This gourmet fall salad can be made up to several hours in advance. Let it sit at room temperature to blend the flavours.

2 cups fennel, thinly julienned

2 cups apples, thinly julienned

1 Tbs. lemon zest

2 Tbs. lemon juice

2 1/2 Tbs. olive oil

1 Tbs. fresh thyme, minced
 (or 1 tsp. dried thyme)

1 tsp. Celtic sea salt

cracked black pepper, to taste

1/2 cup coarsely chopped walnuts

1. To julienne apple and fennel, slice thinly in one direction and then slice in opposite direction to create matchsticks.

3. In a medium-sized bowl, toss together all salad ingredients except walnuts. Let marinate at room temperature up to 4 hours. Top with walnuts just before serving.

4. Keeps well in the fridge for a couple of days.

Serves 4 to 6

MANY OF THE RAW SALADS THAT FOLLOW ARE MEALS IN THEMSELVES IF EATEN IN SUFFICIENT QUANTITIES, PERHAPS WITH A SOUP, OR A BOWL OF STEAMED GRAINS LIKE RICE AND QUINOA, OR STEAMED VEGETABLES IN SEASON. REMEMBER TO CHOP RAW VEGETABLES FINELY IN ORDER TO ABSORB DRESSING AND TO EASE UP ON THE DEMANDS OF CHEWING!

Arame-Yam Salad   Ⓛ Ⓖ Ⓓ Ⓣ

All seaweeds are exceptional sources of a vast array of minerals. This salad offers the goodness of seaweed in combination with flavours that make it more palatable to those who, like me, don't naturally enjoy that fishy quality. You can also enjoy this salad with hijiki instead of arame.

DRESSING:

1 tsp. cold pressed sesame oil

1 tsp. toasted sesame oil (or use
1 more tsp. cold pressed sesame oil)

1 Tbs. tamari

2 tsp. rice wine vinegar or lemon juice

2 tsp. grated ginger

1 tsp. maple syrup

pinch cinnamon or five-spice powder

VEGETABLES:

1 cup arame,
soaked for 30 minutes and rinsed

2 cups grated yam or sweet potato

1 green onion, chopped

2 inches (5 cm.) daikon radish, grated
– or finely chop a few red radishes

1. Prepare dressing in the bottom of a medium-sized serving bowl
2. Drain seaweed and rinse in a medium-sized colander. Place seaweed in a small serving bowl and gently toss with remaining ingredients. Adjust seasoning and allow to sit at room temperature for 1 hour if possible (for flavours to blend).

Serves 4

Cabbage (or Broccoli) Delight

This salad is basic fare but very special in its own right. It has become one of my personal favourite raw meals. Notice the six flavours that make up a satisfying combination. Sweet: carrot, honey, apple, currants. Sour: apple, vinegar. Salty: celery, Celtic sea salt, cheese. Bitter: broccoli, cabbage, parsley. Astringent: apple, broccoli, cabbage, walnuts. Pungent: onion, cabbage.

DRESSING:

2 Tbs. apple cider vinegar
1 1/2 Tbs. olive oil
1 1/2 Tbs. hemp oil or flax oil
1 Tbs. honey
1 to 2 tsp. Celtic sea salt
1/2 tsp. ground fennel

VEGETABLES:

2 cups green cabbage or broccoli, chopped medium fine
3/4 cup red cabbage, chopped medium fine
1/4 cup sweet onion, finely chopped
1 rib celery, finely sliced
1 carrot, quartered lengthwise and sliced
1/2 cup fresh parsley, chopped
1 apple, cored and diced small
1/2 cup currants or raisins
1/2 cup pecans or walnuts, chopped – or 3 Tbs. pumpkin seeds
1/2 cup raw cheese, diced small (optional)

1. Combine dressing ingredients in the bottom of a large salad bowl.

2. Add vegetables and toss to combine.

3. Keeps well in the fridge for a couple of days.

Serves 4 to 6

Carrot-Beet Salad Ⓛ Ⓖ Ⓓ Ⓣ

Carrots are one of the richest sources of the antioxidant beta-carotene, which benefits virtually every organ of the body including the liver, the lungs, the kidneys, the spleen-pancreas, the intestines, and the skin. Carrots and beets in combination are helpful for hormone regulation during menopause. Enjoy the earthiness of this simple, beautiful salad.

2 1/2 cups grated carrots

1 1/2 cups grated beets

2/3 cup crumbled feta
   or crumbled firm tofu (optional)

1/2 tsp. seasoned sea salt (Herbamare)
   or regular sea salt

1 1/2 tsp. dill weed

2 Tbs. wine vinegar or lemon juice

1 Tbs. hemp oil or flax oil

1 Tbs. olive oil

1. Combine all ingredients in a bowl up to 1 hour before serving.

Serves 4 to 6

"Illness and suffering are the results of the misdirection of creative energy. They are a part of the creative force however. They do not come from a different source than, say, health and vitality. Suffering is not good for the soul unless it teaches you to stop suffering. That is its purpose."

JANE ROBERTS AS SETH

Chinese Cabbage Salad

A nice fresh Oriental-style salad. Sometimes I add some brown rice or buckwheat soba noodles to this dish to make a satisfying meal.

DRESSING:

1 1/2 Tbs. cold pressed sesame oil
1 Tbs. rice vinegar or lemon juice
1 Tbs. nama shoyu or tamari
1 tsp. freshly grated ginger
1 Tbs. maple syrup or honey or agave syrup

SALAD:

3 cups Chinese cabbage or Nappa, thinly sliced
1/2 cup shredded purple cabbage
1/2 cup grated carrot
1/2 cup fresh parsley or cilantro, chopped
1 cup bean sprouts
3 Tbs. chopped almonds or sunflower seeds
2 green onions, chopped
1 Tbs. sesame seeds

1. Whisk together all dressing ingredients in a large salad bowl.
2. Add salad ingredients and toss just before serving.

Serves 4 to 6

Dandelion-Pear Salad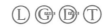

Another gift from Jennifer Italiano of the Live Cafe in Toronto. Surprising and delightful.

DRESSING:

4 Tbs. raw tahini
1 cup orange juice
2 Tbs. dulse flakes
1 Tbs. grated ginger
1/2 tsp. cinnamon
1/2 tsp. curry powder
pinch of salt

1. Blend dressing ingredients in a blender. (A hand blender works well.)
2. Pour over dandelion, pear, onion mixture.
3. Let sit for at least 10 minutes (maximum 2 hours) to marinate.

Serves 4 to 6

SALAD:

1 bunch dandelion, finely chopped
4 pears, thinly sliced
1/2 red onion, thinly sliced

Earth Bowl

This meal is beautiful in its simplicity. It's a satisfying breakfast, lunch or dinner that I really enjoy, made with local ingredients so it's ideal for raw food eating in the colder months.

1 apple, chopped
2 stalks celery, diced
small handful dried currants or raisins or blueberries (or fresh if available)
6 walnuts, broken into pieces
1 Tbs. hemp or pumpkin seeds
juice of 1 orange (optional)

1. Place all ingredients in a bowl and enjoy!

Serves 1

4 F Salad (Favourite, Fast, Flavourful and Filling) Ⓛ Ⓖ Ⓓ Ⓣ

This salad is always great and we eat it often. It's good wrapped in an Ezekiel 4:9 wrap too.

2 avocados

2 Tbs. lemon juice

1 Tbs. olive oil

1/2 Tbs. honey

sea salt, to taste (start with 1 tsp.)

large handful parsley,
  very finely chopped

large handful cilantro,
  very finely chopped

3 green onions, thinly sliced

1 1/2 cups cherry tomatoes, sliced,
  halved, or quartered

Optional: finely chopped red pepper,
  diced cucumber, sauerkraut, sprouts,
  handful finely chopped kale,
  baby salad mix, or arugula

1. In the bottom of a medium-sized bowl, mash 1 avocado with lemon juice, olive oil, honey, and salt.
2. Dice the other avocado and add it to the bowl along with the chopped parsley, cilantro, onions, tomatoes, and other chopped vegetables. Toss gently.
3. Serve on a bed of lettuce and enjoy.

Serves 2 to 4

Kale Avocado Salad Ⓛ Ⓖ Ⓓ Ⓣ

This is a great way to prepare kale, which is highly nutritious but difficult to eat raw for most people who are transitioning to a live foods diet. The kale is massaged with the rest of the ingredients — this wilts the kale and makes it easier on digestion and more palatable. This salad is a staple dish at the Tree of Life, a live foods rejuvenation centre in Arizona. Use any type of kale in this recipe.

1 head kale, thick centre stem removed, finely sliced and then chopped further with a large knife

1 1/2 Tbs. lemon juice

1 tsp. Celtic sea salt

1 avocado, halved, flesh scooped out of peel

1 green onion, thinly sliced

1 tomato, chopped

1. In a large salad bowl, toss together kale, salt, and lemon juice, using your hands to squeeze as you mix (to wilt the kale).

2. Add avocado. Massage into kale until avocado is creamy. Add tomato and green onion, and toss. Serve immediately.

3. As a variation, add chopped fresh herbs, pecans, macadamia, other nuts, or olives.

Serves 2 as a meal, 4 to 6 as a side dish

"To see the world in a grain of sand
And heaven in a wildflower
Hold infinity in the palm of your hand
And eternity in an hour.

He who binds himself to joy
Does the winged life destroy
He who kisses the joy as it flies
Lives in eternity's sunrise."

WILLIAM BLAKE

Dressings and Sauces

Dressings:

Asian Dressing
Avocado Dressing
Balsamic Vinaigrette
Caesar Dressing
Dijon-Miso Dressing
Greek Salad Dressing
Lemon Vinaigrette
Oil-free Dressing
Raspberry Dressing
Sun-dried Tomato Dressing
Tahini Dressing/Dip/Spread
Vinaigrette Dressing

Sauces (and other toppings):

Cheesy Sauce
Cucumber Raita
Ghee
Gomasio
Ketchup à la Raw
Mushroom Sauce
Pine Nut Parmesan
Salsa
Stir-fry Sauce
Tamari Cream Gravy
Teriyaki Sauce and Marinade

Asian Dressing Ⓖ Ⓓ Ⓣ

Use this tasty dressing on your salads for a change. Salad ingredients can include bok choy, nappa, chinese cabbage, broccoli, cauliflower, celery, seaweed, shiitake mushrooms, rice, noodles, baked tofu.

2 Tbs. nama shoyu or tamari

3 Tbs. rice vinegar
 (or cider vinegar is fine)

1 tsp. toasted sesame oil

3 Tbs. raw sesame oil

1 to 2 Tbs. honey or agave syrup

1 clove garlic, minced

1 tsp. (or more) freshly grated
 ginger root, to taste

1. Place all ingredients together in a jar with a tight fitting lid. Shake until combined.

Makes 1/2 cup

THE HEALTHIEST DRESSINGS ARE MADE OF ONLY WHOLE FOOD RAW INGRE-DIENTS. THIS SECTION OFFERS A WIDE RANGE OF DRESSINGS. MANY OF THEM ARE OIL-FREE. IF YOU USE OILS, BE SURE TO CHOOSE COLD PRESSED VERSIONS. MANY DRESS-INGS CAN BE MADE RIGHT IN THE BOTTOM OF THE SALAD BOWL, WHILE OTHERS REQUIRE BLENDING. USE A BLENDER OR HAND-BLENDER, DEPENDING ON QUANTITY.

Avocado Dressing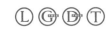

This is a delicious versatile dressing with no added oils. Serve over any garden salad.

1 medium avocado	1. Blend all ingredients until smooth.
1 medium tomato	
1 small celery stalk or 1/2 red pepper	Makes 1 1/2 cups
2 Tbs. lemon juice	
1/2 tsp. salt, to taste	

Balsamic Vinaigrette

An easy, pleasing dressing that uses some of the excellent high quality cold pressed oils available today. To get your family used to the flavours of these oils, you can use half olive oil. This is delicious over fresh organic Boston lettuce or red leaf lettuce, or spring mix.

2 Tbs. cold pressed oil (for example: Udo's Choice, Essential Balance, flax seed oil or hemp oil) – (or use 1/2 olive oil)	1. Combine with a fork in a salad bowl. Add salad ingredients.
1 1/2 Tbs. balsamic vinegar (or for a variation try raspberry wine vinegar)	Makes 1/3 cup, enough a for a large salad (1 head lettuce)
1 Tbs. maple syrup or honey or agave syrup	
1/2 tsp. celtic sea salt	

Caesar Dressing Ⓖ Ⓓ Ⓣ

An egg-free version of a classic.

10 1/2 ounces soft silken tofu	1. Combine all ingredients in blender and process until smooth.
1 Tbs. Dijon mustard	
3 cloves garlic	
1 tsp. Celtic sea salt	Makes 2 cups
1/4 cup olive oil	
1/4 cup fresh lemon juice	
1/4 cup water	
2 tsp. maple syrup	
pepper to taste	
3 Tbs. parmesan cheese (optional)	

Dijon-Miso Dressing Ⓛ Ⓖ Ⓓ Ⓣ

Be sure to use a mild white miso, sometimes called mellow miso, for this dressing.

2 Tbs. white miso	1. By hand, in a small container, mix miso and mustard. Add lemon juice, olive oil, water, and garlic. Whip until well-blended.
2 tsp. Dijon mustard	
4 Tbs. lemon juice	
1/3 cup olive oil	
3 Tbs. water	2. Store in refrigerator in a small covered container.
1 clove garlic, minced	
1 Tbs. honey (optional, for a sweet variation)	Makes 1 cup

Greek Salad Dressing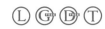

Serve this over various greens (romaine, arugula, spinach), plus cucumber, tomatoes, thinly sliced peppers, thinly sliced red onion, olives and feta.

4 Tbs. olive oil	1. Blend all ingredients until smooth.
2 Tbs. fresh lemon juice	
1/2 tsp. Dijon mustard	Makes 1 cup
1 Tbs. tofu or feta	
1/2 medium tomato	
2 Tbs. water	
1 tsp. Celtic salt	
fresh ground pepper	
4 large basil leaves or 1/2 tsp. dried basil	
1 Tbs. chopped red onion or sweet onion	
1 tsp. red wine vinegar (optional)	

Lemon Vinaigrette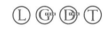

This makes a small jar of dressing, enough for a few large salads. I like to keep it in the fridge for quick salads that I might make for myself for lunch. It's often less daunting to put a salad together if you know the dressing is already made. The olive oil will solidify in the fridge so take the dressing out a half hour before using it.

1/4 cup lemon juice	1. Place ingredients together in a small jar. Shake to combine.
1/4 cup plus 1 Tbs. olive oil	
1 garlic clove, minced	Makes 1/2 cup
1 tsp. honey or agave syrup	
1/2 tsp. sea salt	
pinch thyme and/or oregano and/or basil	

Oil-free Dressing   Ⓛ Ⓖ Ⓓ Ⓣ

This dressing is made from a nut base, in this case walnuts – you could use sunflower seeds too.

3/4 cup walnuts, soaked for 4 hours, then drained and rinsed	1. Blend all ingredients in a blender until smooth.
2 to 3 Tbs. lemon juice	
1 clove garlic	Makes 1 1/2 cups
1 Tbs. chopped red onion or sweet onion	
1/2 cup water (or more), to reach desired consistency	
1 Tbs. mellow miso	
dash nama shoyu or tamari	
pinch Celtic sea salt	
1 Tbs. nutritional yeast (optional)	
1 Tbs. honey (optional)	

Raspberry Dressing   Ⓛ Ⓖ Ⓓ Ⓣ

This oil-free dressing is nice over baby salad greens with chopped fruit such as mango, pineapple, or mandarin oranges.

1 cup raspberries	1. Blend all ingredients until smooth.
juice of 1 orange	
1/4 cup soaked cashews (optional)	Makes 1 1/2 cups
pinch salt (optional)	

Sun-dried Tomato Dressing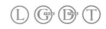

Another oil-free dressing. It's nice served over a fresh salad of tomato, cucumber, red or yellow pepper and fresh chopped basil.

10 sun-dried tomato halves,
   soaked for 1 to 2 hours

1/2 red pepper, chopped

1/4 cup soaked sunflower seeds,
   soaked for 4 hours and drained

tomato soak water, as needed

pinch of salt, to taste (optional)

1. Blend all ingredients together with a blender or hand-blender, adding tomato soak water as needed for required consistency.

Makes 1 cup

Tahini Dressing / Dip / Spread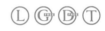

A nutritious versatile recipe. Tahini is made from ground sesame seeds and is high in iron and calcium.

1 1/4 cups raw tahini

1/2 cup (or to taste) lemon juice

1 clove garlic

Celtic sea salt, to taste

1. Mix all ingredients in a bowl until smooth. Store in empty jar.
2. *Dressing:* use 2 Tbs. tahini mixture plus 1 Tbs. water.
3. *Dip:* use 2 Tbs. tahini mixture plus 1/2 Tbs. water.
4. *Spread:* use dip on celery or other vegetables.
5. *Sweeter version:* add honey to taste.

Makes almost 2 cups

Vinaigrette Dressing

A basic yummy recipe for a classic dressing.

| 1/3 cup olive oil |
| 1 Tbs. red wine vinegar |
| 2 Tbs. fresh lemon juice |
| 1/2 tsp. Celtic sea salt |
| 1 Tbs. maple syrup or honey |
| 1 tsp. Dijon mustard |
| fresh herbs (thyme, tarragon, basil), to taste |
| black pepper, to taste |

1. Whisk together all ingredients.

Makes 1/2 cup

THE FOLLOWING SAUCES AND TOPPINGS ADD A LITTLE SOMETHING
SPECIAL TO ANY MEAL. ENJOY!

Cheesy Sauce (L) (G) (D) (T)

I use this sauce for a delicious dairy-free macaroni and cheese.

1 1/2 cups raw cashews
2 cups water
3 Tbs. nutritional yeast
3/4 tsp. (or to taste) salt
1 Tbs. sweet onion
2 Tbs. fresh lemon juice
1 small clove garlic (about 1/2 tsp.)

1. Blend cashews and 1 1/2 cups water in blender until creamy (1 to 2 minutes). Check to be sure there are no cashew pieces remaining.
2. Add and blend the remaining water and all other ingredients.
3. Use over noodles for non-dairy macaroni and cheese (pour over cooked noodles and serve immediately), and/or over steamed vegetables.
4. Refrigerate unused portion.

Makes 3 cups

Cucumber Raita (L) (G) (T)

This is a must with any of the Indian dishes in this book. Fresh and cooling!

1 English cucumber
2 cups organic, non-homogenized (if possible) yogourt
pinch salt
pinch cumin

1. Peel the cucumber if it is non-organic. Grate by hand or with a food processor.
2. Place all ingredients in a medium-sized bowl and stir to combine.

Makes 3 1/2 cups

Ghee Ⓖ Ⓣ

Ghee, also known as clarified butter, is a staple in East Indian cooking. It gives a sweet flavour to vegetables, legumes, and grains and doesn't burn like butter because the milk solids are removed. It doesn't need to be, but can be, refrigerated.

1 lb. organic butter

1. Heat butter over low-medium heat so that it doesn't burn.
2. When it has all melted, begin to skim off all the off-white milk solids that accumulate on top. These milk solids can be spread on toast, tossed with steamed vegetables, or added to soup.
3. Keep heating the butter until it starts to sizzle (do not boil) – this means that all the water has evaporated. Let cool.
4. Store ghee in a wide-mouthed glass jar so that it can be easily spooned out when needed.

Gomasio Ⓛ Ⓖ Ⓓ Ⓣ

Gomasio is a delicious condiment and can be sprinkled on vegetables, salads, and soups. A great way to reduce salt. You can buy it ready-made at the health food store but it's best to make it yourself in small batches so that it's always fresh. Sesame seeds are very high in calcium and iron.

4 Tbs. sesame seeds

1 tsp. sun-dried sea salt

1. Combine and grind in a coffee grinder until fine. Store in a shaker jar.

Makes 1/4 cup

Ketchup à la Raw Ⓛ Ⓖ Ⓓ Ⓣ

Use this delicious condiment on live walnut burgers (see Raw Main Dishes recipes section). We also like it stuffed into avocado halves.

1 cup sun-dried tomatoes
1 cup chopped fresh tomatoes
1 inch (2 1/2 cm.) ginger, chopped
1 tsp. garlic
6 dates
2 Tbs. maple syrup
1 Tbs. apple cider vinegar or lemon juice
8 basil leaves
1 Tbs. nama shoyu or 1 tsp. sea salt
1 Tbs. chopped sweet onion
1/4 cup olive oil

1. Purée all ingredients together in a blender until smooth.
2. Keeps a couple of weeks in the refrigerator.

Makes 2 1/2 cups

In the infinity of life where I am, all is perfect, whole and complete. Change is the natural law of my life. I welcome change. I am willing to change. I choose to change my thinking. I choose to change the words that I use. I move from the old to the new with ease and with joy. LOUISE L. HAY

Mushroom Sauce

This sauce is delicious over patties or savoury loaves. Use rice or quinoa flour for a gluten-free alternative.

1/4 cup chopped leeks or onions	1. Sauté the leeks or onions in butter for 1 minute, then add mushrooms and cook until they are softened.
2 cups chopped mushrooms	
2 Tbs. butter or ghee	2. Add the flour and the yeast, and cook for 1 or 2 more minutes.
2 Tbs. spelt flour or whole wheat flour	
1 tsp. nutritional yeast	3. Gradually pour in the water and then the lemon juice, stirring until the sauce thickens.
1 cup water	
1 tsp. lemon juice (optional)	
1/2 tsp. tarragon	4. Add the herbs and pepper, and cook briefly on low heat to develop the flavours.
1/2 tsp. dill	
pinch of pepper	5. Stir in the tamari and serve. If the sauce gets too thick add a little water or milk, being sure to adjust seasonings.
1 tsp. tamari or Bragg's Liquid Aminos	

Makes about 1 1/4 cups

Pine Nut Parmesan

A nice substitute for those who are avoiding dairy. Sprinkle over any Italian-style dish.

1/2 cup pine nuts	1. Pulse all ingredients in a coffee grinder until coarsely ground.
1/2 tsp celtic sea salt	
1 Tbs. nutritional yeast	Makes 1/2 cup

Salsa Ⓛ Ⓖ Ⓓ Ⓣ

2 cups diced tomatoes
  (1 or 2 or 3 tomatoes)

1/3 cup finely chopped red onion
  or sweet vidalia onion

2 inches (5 cm.) cucumber, diced

palmful of minced cilantro

2 or 3 cloves garlic, minced

1/4 tsp. salt

1/8 tsp. cumin

1/8 tsp. pepper, preferably white

1/4 cup corn niblets (optional)

1/2 cup black beans (optional)

1 tsp. apple cider vinegar

1 tsp. olive oil

1/2 tsp. honey or maple syrup

1. Mix all ingredients together.
2. Refrigerate and let sit up to 24 hours.

Makes 2 1/2 cups

Stir-fry Sauce Ⓖ Ⓓ Ⓣ

1/3 cup tamari

1/3 cup water

2 tsp. fresh grated ginger

1 Tbs. white miso (optional)

1 clove garlic, minced

2 tsp. arrowroot powder

1 tsp. toasted sesame oil

1. Combine all ingredients, except sesame oil, in a bowl.
2. Stir-fry 6 to 8 cups of various vegetables in cold-pressed sesame oil (mushrooms, bean sprouts, celery, carrots, broccoli, zucchini, peppers, onions, etc.) until crisp-tender. Keep in mind cooking time when determining the order in which you cook the vegetables.
3. Immediately add sauce and stir continuously until sauce thickens. Turn off heat and add toasted sesame oil.
4. Serve over brown rice, other grain, or pasta (rice, buckwheat, or udon).

Makes 3/4 cup

"By God, when you see your beauty, you'll be the idol of yourself." RUMI

Tamari Cream Gravy   Ⓣ

A delicious and easy savoury sauce for vegetables, patties, or loaves. You could stir fry leeks and/or mushrooms in the oil before adding the flour. You could also add herbs to taste. I serve this over Shepherd's Pie, Eggplant Patties, Cashew-Carrot Loaf, Grain Patties, and Root Fries.

1 Tbs. olive oil
1 Tbs. butter (or another Tbs. olive oil)

4 Tbs. light spelt flour or
   whole wheat flour
   (or use rice or quinoa flour
   for a gluten-free alternative)

2 cups water
3 Tbs. tamari

1. Gently heat butter and oil over medium heat.
2. Slowly stir in flour, little by little, until it forms a smooth paste. Cook for 1 minute stirring constantly.
3. Still stirring, add water, little by little, to form a smooth thick sauce, using a whisk if necessary.
4. Add tamari, still stirring constantly.
5. Taste and adjust seasoning.
6. After this gravy sits for awhile, you may also have to add a little more water (or any kind of milk). Makes 2 1/2 cups

Teriyaki Sauce and Marinade

Try this marinade on baked or barbecued tofu and vegetables. Good for kebabs. You could also marinate chopped raw vegetables in this sauce for 3 to 4 hours.

1/3 cup tamari (or nama shoyu   if you want to keep it raw)
2 Tbs. water
2 Tbs. freshly squeezed lemon juice
1 Tbs. pure maple syrup or agave syrup
1 Tbs. cold pressed sesame oil
2 tsp. finely grated ginger
1 clove garlic, minced
1 tsp. toasted sesame oil (optional)

1. Put all ingredients into a large jar; cover with the lid and shake until mixed.

Makes 3/4 cup

"God wrote not the laws in the pages of books,

but in your heart and in your spirit.

They are in your breath, your blood, your bone; in your flesh,

your bowels, your eyes, your ears, and in every little part of your body.

They are present in the air, in the water, in the earth, in the plants,

in the sunbeams, in the depths and in the heights.

They all speak to you that you may understand the tongue

and the will of the living God."

THE ESSENE GOSPEL OF PEACE

Cooked Main Dishes

Baked Tofu Fingers
Boston Baked Beans
Brown Moon Curry
Cashew-Carrot Loaf
Cauliflower, Spinach, and Potato
 with Coconut Cream
Chili
Cilantro Tempeh
Dahl
East Indian Peas and Tofu
Eggplant Patties
Enchiladas
Grain Patties
Kitchari
Lentils and Rice
Lentil Chili
Macrobiotic Combo
Meal in a Wrap
Pasta with Beans and Greens
Potato Cauliflower Curry
Rice with Nuts and Raisins
Shepherd's Pie
Spaghetti Sauce
Spicy Tofu with Apricots
Spinach and Sun-dried Tomato Pasta Sauce
Sweet and Sour Tofu and Vegetables
Tacos
Thai Peanut Stir-fry
Tofu Cacciatore
Vegetarian Stew
White Bean Sauce for Pasta

Baked Tofu Fingers

Simple, yummy, and a kid pleaser. Tofu, eaten in moderation, is an excellent vegan source of protein and calcium. Make sure you buy a firm tofu made from organic, non-genetically-modified soybeans. You can also make this recipe with the Teriyaki Sauce and Marinade.

1 lb. firm or extra firm tofu
2 Tbs. tamari
1 Tbs. olive oil or cold-pressed sesame oil

1. Preheat oven to 350F.
2. Slice tofu in half lengthwise and then cut these two halves into 1/4 inch (1/2 cm.) thick slices.
3. Mix oil and tamari in an 8 inch x 14 inch glass pan and dip each piece of tofu into sauce, coating it well.
4. Arrange tofu in the same pan in a single layer. Bake for 25 to 35 minutes depending on how crispy you like it, turning slices once halfway through cooking time.

Serves 4

Boston Baked Beans

The original version of this recipe comes from May All Be Fed, by John Robbins. If you like baked beans, you'll love this recipe. I often double it and freeze in meal-sized portions. To make beans more digestible, follow soaking, rinsing, and cooking directions carefully and then at mealtime, combine with fresh vegetables rather than starches.

2 cups navy beans, picked over and rinsed
1 medium onion, finely chopped
2 tsp. olive oil
1/3 cup fruit-sweetened ketchup
1/4 cup unsulphured molasses
3 Tbs. tamari
3 Tbs. maple syrup
1 Tbs. dry mustard
1 tsp. sea salt

1. Put beans in a large bowl and add enough water to cover by 2 inches (5 cm.). Put the bowl in a cool place and let the beans soak for 12 to 18 hours. Drain and rinse the beans.
2. Put the beans in a large pot and add enough fresh water to cover by 2 inches (5 cm.). Cover and bring to a boil over medium-high heat, then immediately reduce the heat and simmer until the beans are tender (1 1/2 to 2 hours, depending on the age of the beans).
3. Drain the beans, reserving the cooking liquid. Put the beans in a 2-quart baking dish.
4. Preheat the oven to 325F.
5. In a large skillet, sauté the onion in oil until softened (about 10 minutes). If necessary to prevent sticking, add water.
6. Stir the onions into the beans along with the remaining ingredients. Add enough of the cooking liquid to barely cover the beans.
7. Bake covered for 2 to 3 hours, adding cooking liquid when necessary, until beans are nicely browned. Serve hot.
8. Alternatively, I have cooked these beans at 225F overnight for 8 hours.

Serves 8

Brown Moon Curry

An adaptation of a Vegetarian Times recipe contest winner. Yummy!

RICE:

2 cups long-grain brown rice
(brown Jasmine or Basmati are good too)

4 cups water

1 Tbs. curry powder

1 tsp. minced ginger

1/2 tsp. salt

VEGETABLES AND SAUCE:

2 medium sweet potatoes, peeled
and sliced 1/2 inch (1 cm.) thick

3 cups fresh spinach, stems removed,
chopped coarsely

1 red bell pepper, cored and diced

1 1/2 cups sliced fresh mushrooms

3 cloves garlic, minced

1/2 tsp. fresh ginger

1 Tbs. coconut oil, ghee, or olive oil

1 cup coconut milk

1 to 2 tsp. Thai chili sauce

3/4 cup water

1/2 cup whole basil leaves, sliced thinly,
divided (reserve 5 leaves for garnish)

1 cup peeled and chopped fresh pineapple

salt, to taste

CONDIMENTS:

Toasted unsalted organic peanuts or
raw almonds, coarsely chopped

Unsweetened coconut flakes

1 large banana, sliced

lemon juice as needed

1/4 cup raisins

PREPARATION TIME: 45 MINUTES

1. Put rice, water, curry powder, ginger, and salt into a medium-sized saucepan. Bring to a boil. Simmer 30 to 40 minutes until water is absorbed. Turn off heat and let sit.

2. Meanwhile, steam sweet potatoes about 10 minutes (or until barely tender). If you are using a steamer basket, layer potatoes in bottom of basket and lay spinach on top until barely wilted, or quickly steam spinach in a separate pot. Plunge spinach into cold water, then drain. Roll spinach into balls; squeeze dry, and chop coarsely. Set aside.

3. In a large skillet or wok over medium heat, sauté red pepper, mushrooms, garlic, and ginger in oil for approximately 5 minutes. Add coconut milk, chili sauce, and water.

4. Cook uncovered, over medium heat until sauce is heated through. Add sweet potatoes and cook until tender. During the final minute add spinach, basil (except 5 leaves cut into thin ribbons for garnish), and pineapple and heat through. Add salt to taste.

5. Transfer rice to a large serving platter; top with curry and basil ribbons. Serve with condiments on the side.

Serves 6 to 8

Cashew-Carrot Loaf

This loaf is excellent served with Tamari Cream Gravy, roasted potatoes, or various in-season vegetables and big green salad. A delicious feast-day food!

6 cups chopped carrots
2 cups ground cashews
2 Tbs. olive oil
1 cup finely chopped leeks or mild onions
1 cup finely chopped celery
1/2 cup flour (whole wheat, spelt, oat, rice or quinoa)
1 tsp. sea salt
1/2 tsp. black pepper
2 tsp. crushed sage
1/2 tsp. thyme
1 tsp. basil

PREPARATION TIME: 30 MINUTES

1. Steam carrots until tender, then mash them (using a fork, potato masher, blender, or food processor). Six cups of chopped raw carrots make approximately 3 cups mashed.
2. Grind the cashews in a food processor or blender until they are quite fine.
3. Mix all ingredients together and place in an oiled loaf pan.
4. Bake at 350F for 35 to 45 minutes or until the top edges begin to look dry.
5. Cut into squares and serve.

Serves 8

Cauliflower, Spinach, and Potato with Coconut Cream ⓖⓓ

A heavenly dish — what more can I say?

1/2 lb. potatoes,
   sliced 1/3 inch (1 cm.) thick

1 small cauliflower, cut into small florets

5 green onions, sliced including a
   few inches of the greens

1/2 cup chopped cilantro

1/2 tsp. turmeric

2 serrano chilis, minced
   (or use a dash of hot sauce)

one 15-ounce can unsweetened
   coconut milk

1 Tbs. coconut oil

1 large bunch spinach or
   3 cups baby spinach

1/2 tsp. salt

PREPARATION TIME: 30 MINUTES

1. Steam the potatoes in a steamer
basket for 5 minutes, add cauliflower,
steam 5 more minutes until tender,
and remove from heat.

2. Set aside 2 Tbs. each of the green
onions and cilantro, and

3. Puree the remaining green onion,
cilantro, turmeric, chili, and coconut
milk in a blender.

4. Heat a wok or a large skillet and
then add the coconut oil. When hot,
add the green onions and stir-fry for
1 minute.

5. Add the spinach and stir-fry until
wilted and tender.

6. Pour in the coconut mixture. Add
the cauliflower and potatoes, season
with 1/2 tsp. salt, and simmer until
heated through.

7. Taste and adjust seasoning. Serve
garnished with the reserved cilantro.

Serves 4

Chili Ⓖ Ⓓ Ⓣ⁺

When making this for fussy eaters, chop all the vegetables very finely in a food processor so that they are hidden in the chili and can't be picked out by little fingers! My students tell me that this chili kicks! It's mildly spiced so add more cayenne or hot sauce if you prefer a fiery chili.

3 cups dried kidney beans, picked over and rinsed – or 2 large cans kidney beans, drained and rinsed thoroughly

2 Tbs. olive oil or coconut oil

2 onions, finely chopped

1 celery stalk with leaves, finely chopped

1 medium carrot, finely chopped

1 red pepper, finely chopped

1 cup mushrooms, sliced

6 cloves garlic, minced

2 Tbs. chili powder

2 tsp. cumin

2 Tbs. dried parsley

2 bay leaves

2 tsp. dried oregano

1/8 tsp. (or more) cayenne pepper, to taste

1 tsp. (or to taste) salt

one 28-ounce can crushed tomatoes

2 to 5 1/2 cans tomato paste

1 to 2 cups vegetable broth, water, or bean cooking liquid (to desired consistency)

1 1/2 cups frozen or fresh corn (optional)

2 Tbs. apple cider vinegar or red wine vinegar

1 Tbs. honey

2 Tbs. tamari

PREPARATION TIME: 40 MINUTES

1. Put the beans in a bowl and add enough water to cover by 2 inches (5 cm.). Let soak for at least 8 hours (maximum 24 hours). Drain and rinse thoroughly. Put the beans in a medium-sized pot, cover with 2 inches (5 cm.) of fresh water (add a strip of kombu if desired – said to reduce gas-causing effects). Bring to a boil, reduce the heat to low and simmer, covered, for 1 1/2 to 2 hours until the beans are tender (you should be able to mash them easily on the roof of your mouth). Stir occasionally. Drain the beans, reserving liquid. Or use 2 large cans of beans, drained and rinsed thoroughly.

2. In a large pot gently stir fry onions, celery, carrots, garlic, mushrooms, and green pepper in oil, over medium heat, until softened (7 to 10 minutes). If necessary to prevent sticking, add water.

3. Add the spices and herbs and cook on low for 5 minutes, stirring often.

4. Add the tomatoes, tomato paste, beans, and vegetable stock and cook for another 40 minutes, until thickened.

5. Stir in the corn, vinegar, honey, and tamari, cook 5 minutes and adjust seasonings. Remove bay leaves before serving.

Serves 6 to 8
(can be doubled and frozen)

Cilantro Tempeh Ⓖ Ⓓ Ⓣ⁺

Tempeh is arguably the best way to enjoy soybeans as they are fermented and therefore more digestible. Umeboshi vinegar is a Japanese condiment often used in macrobiotic cooking. You can buy it at the health food store (along with the tempeh!). Jacqueline who doesn't usually like cilantro loves this dish and takes some to school the next day if there are leftovers.

1 package tempeh (225g)

2 cups water

2 Tbs. sesame oil

1 cup sweet onion, sliced

1/2 tsp. coriander

1/2 tsp. cumin

2 tsp. crushed garlic

1/4 tsp. cayenne pepper

1/2 cup water

3 Tbs. umeboshi vinegar

1/2 cup cilantro, chopped

1/3 cup red pepper, chopped

3/4 - 1 cup chopped tomato

salt, to taste (sometimes the vinegar already has salt so taste first)

PREPARATION TIME: 15 MINUTES

1. Boil tempeh in water for 10 minutes. When cool, cut into small dice-sized cubes and set aside.
2. Heat oil in a skillet, add onions and cook on medium heat for 5 minutes.
3. Add coriander, cumin, garlic, cayenne and cook another couple of minutes.
4. Add tempeh and water and cook over low-medium heat for 15 more minutes.
5. Add umeboshi vinegar, cilantro, pepper and tomato. Heat through, salt to taste and serve.

Serves 4

Dahl Ⓖ Ⓓ Ⓣ

Dahl simply means legumes in East Indian. It is difficult to plan healthy meatless meals without using legumes in some form or another. In Ayurvedic medicine, it is said that we should be eating legumes at least once a day, not necessarily in large quantities. The key to preparing legumes that are delicious, flavourful, and easily digested is cooking them correctly with spices and, in the case of this recipe, ghee (see Dressings and Sauces). Dahl can be eaten as a side dish, spooned over rice and/or vegetables, or it can be used as a dip for bread. Only a small amount of dahl (usually less than 1/2 cup) is necessary to balance out a meal. Leftovers can be thinned out with water or vegetable broth for a lovely soup. This dahl is nice served with rice, Raita (cucumbers and yogourt), and Potato Cauliflower Curry for an Indian-style meal.

---

2 cups split peas (yellow or green), lentils (brown or red), or mung beans (soaked overnight)

water, enough to create a thick soupy consistency

2 to 3 Tbs. ghee (clarified butter-see Dressings and Sauces) or coconut oil

3/4 Tbs. turmeric

1 1/2 Tbs. cumin

2 1/2 Tbs. coriander

1 large onion, sliced or finely chopped

mushrooms, sliced (optional)

green pepper, sliced

1 1/2 tsp. sea salt

---

1. Wash legumes taking care to discard pebbles and defective beans.
2. Place legumes in a large pot and add water until it is 2 inches (5 cm.) above the legumes.
3. Bring to a boil and cook over low-medium heat until beans are tender. This will vary depending on the age and type of legume (15 minutes for red lentils, up to 40 minutes for some of the other legumes). Add water when necessary to maintain a thick soupy consistency.
4. Meanwhile, in a heavy skillet (cast iron works well) heat ghee over medium heat. Add turmeric, cumin, and coriander until browned, being careful not to burn the spices.
5. Next, add to this the sliced onions until golden, followed by any of the optional vegetables, cooked until soft.
6. When the legumes are very soft (there should be no hint of a crunch!), add them to the vegetables in the skillet (if it is large enough – otherwise add the vegetables to the legumes) and cook for 10 to 15 minutes, again adding water if necessary to maintain a soupy mixture.
Makes 5 to 6 cups

East Indian Peas and Tofu

A delicious, flavourful, non-dairy alternative to peas paneer. Garam masala is a classic Indian spice mixture that can be bought at specialty stores and Indian grocers.

500 grams tofu, quartered lengthwise and sliced 1/2 inch (1 cm.) thick

2 Tbs. ghee or coconut oil

1 tsp. cumin seeds

4 green cardamoms, skinned

1 inch (2 1/2 cm.) cinnamon

1 cup chopped leek or onion

1 tsp. mustard seeds

1 tsp. poppy seeds

1 inch (2 1/2 cm.) ginger, grated

1 tsp. turmeric

1/2 tsp. paprika

2 cups peas, fresh or frozen

4 tomatoes, chopped

2 cups water

1 tsp. salt

1 tsp. garam masala

1 Tbs. lemon juice

PREPARATION TIME: 30 MINUTES

1. In a medium-sized saucepan, fry tofu in 1 Tbs. ghee until golden brown. Remove from pan and set aside.

2. Grind cumin seeds, cardamom, and cinnamon using a coffee grinder or a mortar and pestle.

3. Fry leek (or onion) in remaining ghee until soft.

4. Add mustard seeds and poppy seeds and fry for 1 minute.

5. Add ginger, turmeric, paprika, plus ground cumin, cardamom, and cinnamon and fry for 2 more minutes.

6. Add peas, tomatoes, water, tofu, and salt and simmer for 10 minutes until heated through.

7. Just before serving, add garam masala and lemon juice. Taste and adjust salt.

Serves 6

Eggplant Patties

Most people love these even though they may not normally like eggplant. Serve with Tamari Cream Gravy.

1 large eggplant skin on, washed and cubed (crouton size, 7 to 8 cups)

3/4 cup water

2/3 cup ground walnuts or cashews (or use a mixture – sometimes I use hazelnuts or pecans as well)

2 slices whole grain bread

1/3 cup finely chopped celery

3/4 cup rolled oats

1/2 tsp. salt or Herbamare

3/4 tsp. sage

1 Tbs. tamari

PREPARATION TIME: 30 MINUTES

1. Place eggplant and water in a medium-sized saucepan, bring to a boil and simmer for 10 minutes until eggplant is tender. Drain and mash eggplant.
2. Meanwhile, process nuts, bread and celery in a food processor until finely ground. Add rolled oats and pulse a few times.
3. Add this mixture to the eggplant as well as seasoning. Mix well. Let stand for 5 minutes.
4. Shape into patties and place on a lightly oiled cookie sheet.
5. Bake at 350F for 12 minutes, turn and bake 10 minutes more until patties are firm and crisp, but still moist on the inside.

Makes approximately 12 patties (can be doubled and frozen)

Enchiladas ⓢ

These tasty rolls are adapted from the Salt Spring Island Cookbook. Every year the teenagers at the Ashtanga Yoga Fellowship Retreat beg me to make these, and so we end up making a couple hundred of them. Late at night they sneak into the huge walk-in fridge to snack on leftovers.

3 cups cooked red kidney beans or pinto beans (from about 1 1/2 cups dry) – Or two 14-ounce cans kidney beans or pinto beans

1 cup finely chopped leeks or onions

1 cup finely chopped red or green pepper

2 Tbs. olive oil

1 tsp. sea salt

3 Tbs. chili powder

1/4 tsp. cayenne or a couple of dashes of hot sauce, to taste

4 Tbs. liquid from cooking the beans

2 Tbs. lemon juice

1 1/2 tsp. cumin

SAUCE:

2 Tbs. chili powder

1/2 cup corn meal

1/2 tsp. sea salt

4 Tbs. light spelt flour

3 Tbs. olive oil

24 ounces crushed tomatoes

8 to 10 tortilla wraps (whole wheat, spelt, or preferably sprouted grain (Ezekiel 4:9))

grated cheese

salsa, guacamole, and yogourt or sour cream (for garnish)

PREPARATION TIME: 30 MINUTES

1. If using beans from dry, soak beans overnight and then rinse thoroughly and drain.

2. Add fresh water and cook until tender, approximately 1 1/2 to 2 1/2 hours.

3. In a large, heavy skillet sauté leeks or onions in oil until they are just tender. Combine with the remaining ingredients in a large bowl. Mix thoroughly.

4. Make sauce: In a saucepan, sauté the chili powder, salt, cornmeal, and flour in the oil for 1 to 2 minutes. Then add tomatoes and simmer for approximately 10 minutes, stirring occasionally. If necessary add water to the sauce so that it is thick and will pour easily over the enchiladas.

5. Put 2 to 3 Tbs. of filling in a line across the middle of each tortilla. Roll up tortillas and place them seam side down on an oiled 8 inch x 12 inch baking dish. A cookie sheet can work fine too.

6. Pour sauce over prepared enchiladas, top with grated cheese if desired, and bake for 20 to 25 minutes at 325F.

7. Garnish with salsa, guacamole, and yogourt or sour cream.

Serves 4 to 6

Grain Patties

A good way to get your family and friends accustomed to whole grains. You can use any combination of grains for these patties. Or use just millet or just rice. For a fall or winter meal, I like to serve them with Tamari Cream Gravy, mashed or roasted potatoes or Root Fries, steamed vegetables, and a big salad. They're also nice on a bun or stuffed into a pita with lettuce or sprouts, tomatoes, pickles, ketchup, mustard, and other condiments.

1/4 cup millet

1/4 cup brown rice (short grain is stickier)

1/4 cup barley

1 3/4 cups water

1/2 lb. medium firm tofu (225 grams)

1/2 cup sunflower seeds, ground
(a coffee grinder works well)

1/2 cup finely chopped onion or leek

1 cup grated carrot

1 cup coarse bread crumbs or rolled oats

1 Tbs. tamari

1 Tbs. nutritional yeast

1 tsp. thyme

1 tsp. sage

2 tsp. dill

1/2 tsp. (or to taste) sea salt

1/2 tsp. pepper

3 Tbs. olive oil

PREPARATION TIME: 40 MINUTES

1. Wash grains and drain. Place in medium-sized pot with water and bring to a boil. Turn heat down, cover, and simmer 45 minutes. Allow to cool.

2. Add remaining ingredients, mix thoroughly (I use my hands), and form into patties. You can also run the entire mixture through a meat grinder or masticating juicer. Test to be sure that burgers will hold together well – if not, add a little spelt flour or more oats.

3. Bake at 325F on greased baking sheet for 15 minutes, flip and cook for another 15 minutes.

Makes approximately 12 patties
(recipe can be doubled and frozen)

Kitchari ⒼⒹⓉ⁺

This is a mildly spiced simple Indian stew that is balancing and protein packed. Mung beans are the easiest legume to digest and in this recipe they are soaked along with the rice. Enjoy it with a dollop of yogourt.

1 cup brown rice (soaked 8 hours) –
long-grain or brown basmati

1/2 cup whole mung beans
(soaked 8 hours)

2 Tbs. ghee or coconut oil

1 large onion sliced fine

1 garlic clove, minced

2 tsp. ginger, grated or minced

1/4 tsp. ground cloves

1/2 tsp. turmeric

3/4 tsp. cinnamon

1/2 tsp. cardamom

handful cilantro, chopped

7 or 8 mint leaves, chopped

2 tomatoes or 1 14 oz can diced tomatoes

3 cups water

1 - 2 tsp. salt, to taste

2 cups chopped cauliflower (and/or
other vegetables like green beans
or potatoes)

1. Soak brown rice and mung beans together for about 8 hours, drain and rinse.

2. In a large pot, heat ghee or coconut oil and fry onions, garlic, ginger and spices gently for about 7 minutes.

3. Add cilantro, mint and tomatoes, stirring for about 3 minutes.

4. Add drained rice, mung beans, water and salt. Cook on medium low heat for 40 minutes.

5. Add cauliflower and other vegetables if desired and simmer for 8 to 10 more minutes until vegetables are tender and rice is quite soft, adding more water as necessary.

Serves 6

Lentils and Rice

Quick, economical, healthy, and good — what more could you want? Serve with a large salad and a steamed vegetable. The secret to this recipe is to allow the onions to gently fry until golden brown.

3/4 cup brown rice

1 1/2 cups water

2/3 cup dried brown lentils or
    green lentils

3 cups water

2 large onions, finely chopped
    (or use leeks)

3 Tbs. olive oil

1 tsp. salt

1. Place rice and 1 1/2 cups water in a pot with a tight-fitting lid, bring to a boil and then reduce heat to minimum for 20 minutes. Turn off heat and allow rice to stand for another 15 minutes.

2. Place lentils and 3 cups water in a medium-sized pot. Bring to a boil, then reduce heat to medium-low until lentils are tender but still firm (approximately 25 to 25 minutes).

3. Meanwhile, in a large skillet, stir-fry onions in olive oil over medium heat to start then reducing to low, until onions are well-browned.

4. Add lentils and rice to onions, plus salt, and toss to combine.

Serves 4

Lentil Chili Ⓖ Ⓓ Ⓣ⁺

This delicious sauce can be stuffed into a steamed whole wheat pita or served over brown rice.

4 cups lentils (brown, green, or red)

6 to 7 cups water (2 of these can be tomato juice if desired)

one 18-ounce can tomatoes or use the equivalent in fresh tomatoes

2 tsp. ground cumin

1 tsp. paprika

1/2 tsp. dried thyme

10 (yes 10!) medium-sized cloves garlic, minced

2 medium onions, finely chopped

1 to 2 tsp. salt, to taste

lots of fresh black pepper

one 5 1/2-ounce can tomato paste

1 1/2 Tbs. red wine vinegar or balsamic vinegar

crushed red pepper (or anything else that will make it the desired hotness), to taste

1. Place lentils and 6 cups water in a large pot. Bring to boil, partially cover, and simmer for 30 minutes.

2. Add tomatoes, cumin, paprika, thyme, garlic, and onions. Stir and let cook for 45 to 60 minutes, stirring from the bottom every 10 to 15 minutes, until lentils are tender. To prevent dryness, check water level as it cooks and add water in 1/4 cup increments as needed.

3. Add salt, pepper, and tomato paste. Stir and continue to simmer slowly, partially covered, until the lentils are very soft (maximum another 30 minutes).

4. Add vinegar and red pepper. Taste, adjust seasonings, and serve. Freezes well.

Serves at least 8

Macrobiotic Combo

This is a very nice winter meal which follows classic macrobiotic principles.

NAVY BEAN STEW:

1 cup navy beans, soaked overnight

4 inches (10 cm.) kombu (optional, but said to aid in digestion of beans)

1 Tbs. olive oil

1 medium onion, diced

1 celery stalk, cut in half lengthwise then in 1/4 inch (1/2 cm.) slices

1 medium carrot, cut in half then in 1/2 inch (1 cm.) diagonal slices

1 tsp. sea salt

1/2 cup chopped parsley

MILLET:

1 1/2 cups millet

3 cups water

VEGETABLES:

1 bunch kale, stems removed, sliced in 3/4 inch (2 cm.) strips

2 cups cubed yams (1 or 2 yams)

MISO GRAVY:

1 Tbs. miso

1/3 cup water

1 Tbs. cold-pressed sesame oil (not toasted)

1 cup chopped leeks (or sweet onions)

3 Tbs. spelt flour

1/2 tsp. dried thyme

1 1/2 cups water

1 Tbs. tamari

PREPARATION TIME: 45 MINUTES

1. *Navy bean stew:* Drain soaked beans, cover with fresh water by 2 inches (5 cm.), add kombu, and bring to a boil. Earlier in the day, simmer and cook beans for 1 hour, until beans are almost tender. Then heat oil in a medium-sized pot and gently fry onion, then celery, then carrots, until vegetables have wilted. Add cooked beans with liquid, salt, and parsley. Simmer 30 minutes, or until beans are fully cooked.

2. *Millet:* Wash and drain millet in a medium-sized pot. Add fresh water and bring to a boil. Turn heat down to low and simmer for 40 minutes. Turn off heat and let sit.

3. *Vegetables:* Place prepared vegetables in a steamer basket and steam until tender, approximately 12 to 15 minutes.

4. *Miso gravy:* In a cup, mix miso and water to form a smooth paste and set aside. Heat oil in a pot, add leeks and gently fry for approximately 5 minutes. Add flour and thyme, stirring constantly until combined and smooth. Slowly add water, stirring with a wire whisk, allowing the mixture to boil gently until thick. Add tamari, turn off heat, and add miso mixture. Taste and adjust.

5. *To serve:* Spread a spoonful of millet on each individual plate. Then vegetables on top, beans on the side, and gravy over everything. Sprinkle with gomasio (sesame seed salt – see Dressings and Sauces)

Serves 4 or 5

Meal in a Wrap   Ⓢ Ⓓ Ⓣ

This is a quick fun meal – place all ingredients on the table and let people put their own wraps together. Children will eat what they make for themselves.

legumes (leave whole or mash with
  salt and chili powder):
  black beans
  pinto beans
  refried beans
  (you can even buy these beans canned
  and seasoned at the health food store)

barbecued onions (fry until soft and
  then add natural barbecue sauce)

fresh vegetables:

chopped tomatoes

shredded lettuce

chopped green onions

sliced red onions

thinly sliced red or green peppers

asparagus spears, lightly steamed

sprouts

shredded carrots

shredded cheese

olives

guacamole

salsa

1. Wrap Ezekiel wraps or whole wheat tortillas in a damp towel and place in a large casserole in oven at 150F for approximately 20 minutes.
2. Meanwhile, prepare bowls of various stuffings and place on table.

Pasta with Beans and Greens

Pasta fagioli. An Italian peasant dish fit for royalty. A meal in a bowl. Serve with a fresh salad or raw vegetables. Like many of the recipes in this book, this recipe has all of the 6 flavours needed to nourish our bodies and our souls. Sweet pasta, spicy garlic, astringent beans, sour lemon, bitter greens, and salt.

1 cup dried romano beans or use one
   14-ounce can romano beans
   (white kidney beans work well too)

1 pound short chunky pasta
   (rice or kamut)

3 Tbs. minced garlic

1 1/2 cups diced onions or leeks

2 Tbs. olive oil

1 bunch spinach or chard (broccoli or
   rapini are good too)

salt and pepper

3 cups chopped fresh tomatoes or one
   28-ounce can diced tomatoes

juice of 1 lemon

PREPARATION TIME: 30 MINUTES

1. If using dry beans, soak overnight, then rinse well. Place in pot and cover with 2 inches (5 cm.) water. Bring to a boil, then turn down heat, cover and simmer until very tender (approximately 1 hour).

2. Bring a large covered pot of water to a rapid boil.

3. While the pasta water heats, in a large-sized saucepan sauté the garlic and onion in 1 Tbs. olive oil until the onion is translucent. Add water if necessary to prevent sticking.

4. Wash and coarsely chop the greens. Stir the greens, salt, and pepper into the onions and cook for several minutes, until the greens are wilted (chard will take a little longer than spinach).

5. When the pasta water boils, stir in the pasta, cover and return to a boil. Cook until al dente.

6. Meanwhile, add the tomatoes and drained beans to the greens and onions and bring the sauce to a simmer. Add the lemon juice just before serving. Add the last Tbs. olive oil. Season with salt and pepper to taste.

7. Serve sauce ladled onto bowls of hot pasta, topped with freshly grated parmesan if desired. Or use Pinenut Parmesan.

Serves 4 to 6

Potato Cauliflower Curry

Every year at the end of the summer, I cooked for the Ashtanga Yoga Retreat at Shadow Lake. One of the challenges, besides cooking for 120 people, is that I couldn't use garlic and onions because they are found by some people to be overly stimulating and not conducive to the meditative experience. Saturday night was always Indian Feast night. I adapted this recipe from the Green Door Restaurant in Ottawa, replacing the onions and garlic with leeks. Garam masala is a mixture of spices found at Indian food stores.

3 Tbs. ghee or coconut butter or olive oil

1/4 tsp. ground cardamom

1/4 tsp. cayenne

1/2 tsp. turmeric

1/2 tsp. ground cumin

1 tsp. garam masala

1 cup chopped leeks

1 small head cauliflower, cut into florets

3 medium potatoes,
　cut into medium-sized chunks

1 yam, cut into medium-sized chunks

2 to 3 cups water

salt, to taste

one 15-ounce can unsweetened
　coconut milk (choose the best quality
　with no preservatives)

1/2 red pepper, diced

1/2 green pepper, diced

1 cup diced fresh tomato

1/2 cup chopped fresh coriander

PREPARATION TIME: 30 MINUTES

1. In a medium-sized pot, over medium-low heat melt oil and add spices, stirring, for 1 to 2 minutes. Add leeks and sauté for 5 minutes over medium heat. Add cauliflower and potatoes and sauté for another few minutes.

2. Add salt, coconut milk and just enough water to barely cover the vegetables and cook until vegetables are tender. Add peppers, tomato, and coriander and cook another 5 minutes.

3. Taste, adjust seasoning and serve.

Serves 6 to 8

Rice with Nuts and Raisins

A flavourful way to enjoy rice!

2 Tbs. olive oil
1 1/2 cups finely chopped onion
2 large cloves garlic
1 tsp. minced fresh ginger
2 cups uncooked brown rice (basmati works well)
3 cups boiling water
1 Tbs. butter
1 cup chopped nuts (cashews, walnuts, and/or pecans)
1 cup raisins
1/2 tsp. (or to taste) salt
1/2 to 1 tsp. grated lemon rind or orange rind (or a combination)

PREPARATION TIME: 50 MINUTES

1. Heat the oil in a large-sized saucepan. Add onions, garlic, and ginger, and sauté over medium heat for approximately 5 minutes, stirring frequently.

2. Add the uncooked rice, and continue to sauté with occasional stirring for another 5 to 8 minutes. Meanwhile, boil the water.

3. Pour in the boiling water, cover, and turn the heat down to minimum. Simmer very gently, undisturbed, for 40 minutes. Check for tenderness and if necessary cook for another 5 to 10 minutes.

4. While the rice is simmering, melt the butter in a heavy skillet, add the chopped nuts, and sauté over low-medium heat for 5 minutes until the nuts are lightly browned. Stir in the raisins, salt, and grated lemon rind or orange rind. Cook for 1 more minute, then remove from heat and set aside.

5. When rice is tender, add the nut mixture and mix gently until well combined. Serve hot.

Serves 6

Shepherd's Pie   ⓖ ⓓ

This is a crowd pleaser and a family favourite. Tamari Cream Gravy is a must. Serve with a big fresh salad. Adapted from The Pheylonian Cookbook, by the Chikalos.

3 cups water

1/2 cup millet, washed

1/2 cup quinoa, washed

1/2 cup hulled buckwheat, washed

1/2 tsp. salt

2 Tbs. tamari

1 clove garlic, minced

1 tsp. thyme

1 tsp. coriander

1/2 tsp. sage

1/4 tsp. savory

MIDDLE LAYER:

1 1/2 cups diced leeks or onions

1 Tbs. ghee or olive oil

1 1/2 cups frozen organic corn

1/2 tsp. salt

1 Tbs. natural barbecue sauce (optional)

MASHED POTATOES:

6 to 7 good-sized potatoes,
  peeled and quartered

2 Tbs. butter or olive oil

water or milk (rice, soy, almond, or dairy)

PREPARATION TIME: 60 MINUTES

1. Preheat oven to 350F.

2. Using a large-sized pot, boil water and add millet. Turn heat down and simmer for 20 to 30 minutes, until millet granules appear to be well open and the liquid creamy. Add quinoa and buckwheat, stir and simmer over low heat for 30 minutes.

3. Let cool to room temperature. Crumble this 3-grain mixture in the pot and add tamari, garlic, and herbs, plus salt to taste.

4. Meanwhile, boil quartered potatoes in 4 inches (10 cm.) of water until tender. Drain water and reserve. Mash potatoes, adding butter or oil and cooking water and/or milk until creamy. Add salt to taste.

5. Meanwhile, fry onions in ghee or oil until tender and golden. Add corn, salt and optional barbecue sauce to onion mixture.

6. Press 3-grain mixture into an oiled 9 inch x 9 inch casserole.

7. Layer onion-corn mixture on top of grain.

8. Spread mashed potatoes evenly on top of this and bake at 350F until golden brown (approximately 30 minutes).

9. Serve with gravy.

Serves 6 to 8

Spaghetti Sauce Ⓖ Ⓓ Ⓣ⁺

An excellent vegetable laden savoury sauce. Serve over any kind of pasta.

2 Tbs. olive oil
2 onions, chopped
2 cloves garlic, minced
1/2 lb. mushrooms, sliced
2 zucchinis, halved and sliced
2 to 3 stalks celery, sliced
2 carrots, halved and sliced
1 green pepper, chopped
10 cups peeled and chopped tomatoes – or 28 ounces tomatoes + 16 ounces tomato sauce + 6 ounces tomato paste
3 Tbs. tamari
2 Tbs. honey
2 bay leaves
1 tsp. basil
1/2 tsp. oregano
dash thyme
dash marjoram

1. Gently sauté onions in oil over medium heat until tender. Add garlic and mushrooms, and sauté for 1 more minute.
2. Add remaining ingredients and simmer for 1 hour.

Serves 6 to 8

Spicy Tofu with Apricots

This dish is standard fare in my legumes and tofu cooking class — its complex flavours and textures are very enjoyable. Bring the leftovers to work the next day — it's even delicious at room temperature and the flavours intensify. I serve it with quinoa so that my students can experience a different grain.

SAUCE:

4 Tbs. tamari or soya sauce

1 1/2 Tbs. balsamic vinegar

2 tsp. sesame seeds

2 tsp. curry powder

1 tsp. (or to taste) hot chili oil or
   1 to 2 tsp. (or to taste) chili sauce

1 Tbs. maple syrup

1 Tbs. fresh chives (or 1 tsp. dried)

1 Tbs. fresh parsley (or 1 tsp. dried)

TOFU AND VEGETABLES:

1 lb. extra-firm tofu,
   drained and cubed (dice size)

2 tsp. coconut oil or ghee

2 cloves garlic, minced

1 medium onion, chopped

1 medium carrot, sliced diagonally

1/3 cup chopped dry roasted organic
   peanuts or pecans

1/3 cup chopped dried apricots

1. In a large-sized baking dish, mix together sauce ingredients. Marinate tofu in sauce for at least 5 minutes.

2. Heat oil in wok or large frying pan. Stir-fry remaining ingredients until onion has softened.

3. Add tofu and marinating sauce. Heat until tofu has reached desired consistency (maximum 15 minutes).

4. Serve over steamed rice or quinoa.

To cook quinoa: Rinse 1 cup of quinoa under cold water and drain. Bring quinoa and 2 cups of water to a boil, reduce heat to medium-low and simmer for 20 minutes. Turn off heat and let sit 5 to 10 minutes.

Serves 4 to 6

Spinach and Sun-dried Tomato Pasta Sauce (G)(D)(T)+

Make this hearty dish in 30 minutes or less and bring leftovers to work tomorrow.

1/4 cup sun-dried tomatoes

8 ounces pasta of your choice (try rice spirals)

1 small onion, chopped

3 cloves garlic, minced

2 Tbs. olive oil

8 ounces fresh mushrooms, sliced

2 Tbs. tamari

one 16-ounce can artichoke hearts, drained and chopped

1/4 cup chopped kalamata olives

1/4 cup pine nuts

1 bunch fresh spinach, washed and stems removed

3 ounces feta cheese, crumbled (optional)

1. Soak sun-dried tomatoes in hot water for 30 minutes, then drain. Slice into thin strips.

2. Cook pasta according to package directions.

3. Gently sauté onion and garlic in oil over medium-low heat for 2 to 3 minutes. Add mushrooms and tamari and sauté for another 3 minutes, until vegetables are tender. Add tomatoes, artichoke hearts, olives, and pine nuts and toss. Add spinach, toss, and heat through until spinach is wilted.

4. Toss with pasta. Garnish with optional feta cheese or sprinkle with Pinenut Parmesan. Adjust seasonings.

Serves 4

Sweet and Sour Tofu and Vegetables

One of the great stir-frys. Adapted from May All Be Fed, by John Robbins.

RICE:

2 1/2 cups water

1 1/2 cups long-grain brown rice

TOFU:

1 lb. firm tofu, patted dry and cubed

1 tsp. raw sesame oil

1 Tbs. tamari

VEGETABLES:

1 Tbs. oil (coconut, sesame, or olive)

1 large onion, thinly sliced

1 medium carrot, sliced diagonally
into 1/4 inch (1/2 cm.) thick slices

4 ounces green beans, cut into 3/4 inch
(2 cm.) lengths

1 large red bell pepper, seeded and
sliced into 1/2 inch (1 cm.) strips

6 ounces mushrooms, thinly sliced

1 medium zucchini, sliced into 1/2 inch
(1 cm.) thick rounds

1 cup diced fresh pineapple

SAUCE:

1/2 cup fresh orange juice

2 Tbs. lemon juice

2 Tbs. fruit-sweetened ketchup

2 Tbs. maple syrup

2 Tbs. tamari

1 Tbs. toasted sesame oil

2 1/4 tsp. arrowroot powder

2 1/2 tsp. (or to taste)
finely grated ginger root

PREPARATION TIME: 45 MINUTES

1. In a medium-sized pot, bring water and rice to a boil. Cover and reduce heat to minimum for 30 to 40 minutes, until water is absorbed. Then turn heat off and let rice stand for at least 10 minutes.
2. Meanwhile, toss tofu cubes in raw sesame oil and tamari, and bake in oven until browned, approximately 40 minutes.
3. Wash and chop all vegetables and set aside.
4. In a small bowl, combine sauce ingredients and set aside.
5. In a wok or large-sized shallow pot, heat 1 Tbs. oil over medium-high heat. Add vegetables and stir fry for 3 to 5 minutes until crisp tender, adding water if necessary to prevent sticking.
6. Add the sauce and cook stirring often, until sauce thickens (approximately 2 minutes). Add baked tofu and pineapple. Heat through. Serve over rice

Serves 4

Tacos Ⓖ Ⓓ Ⓣ

Tasty and satisfying! Adapted from Marilyn Diamond's excellent book The American Vegetarian Cookbook. This book was my constant companion in my first years as a vegetarian.

1 small onion, diced

1 small red pepper, diced

2 tsp. coconut oil or olive oil

1 tsp. paprika

1 tsp. cumin

1 tsp. chili powder

4 to 6 Tbs. water

1 lb. firm tofu

2 Tbs. natural ketchup

2 Tbs. natural barbecue sauce

salt, to taste

8 corn tortillas or taco shells (you can get some made without hydrogenated oil at the health food store) – or roll mixture and toppings into an Ezekiel 4:9 wrap

TOPPINGS:

chopped avocado or guacamole

tomatoes

green onions

alfalfa sprouts

shredded lettuce

salsa

1. In a large skillet, sauté onion and red pepper in oil, adding paprika, cumin, and chili powder as vegetables begin to soften. Add water and allow vegetables to cook through.

2. Crumble tofu into skillet, add ketchup and barbecue sauce and stir well. Sauté for 5 minutes. Season to taste with salt, if desired.

3. Spoon into warmed tortillas or shells and serve with toppings.

Serves 4

Thai Peanut Stir-fry

With this simple stir-fry dish, vary the vegetables seasonally and serve with the delectable Thai Peanut Sauce that follows.

6 cups cooked brown rice or quinoa
  (see cooking instructions)

one 16-ounce package firm tofu,
  drained and cubed

2 Tbs. coconut oil or raw sesame oil,
  divided

2 cloves garlic, sliced

2 medium carrots, sliced crosswise

1 medium onion, cubed

2 cups broccoli florets

1/4 small head purple cabbage, shredded

1/4 small head green cabbage, shredded

1 medium red bell pepper, cubed

4 green onions, trimmed and
  sliced crosswise

1 cup snow peas

1/4 cup chopped cilantro

2 Tbs. toasted sesame seeds

THAI PEANUT SAUCE:

1/2 cup organic creamy peanut butter or
  almond butter

1 cup freshly squeezed orange juice

2 Tbs. tamari

1 tsp. toasted sesame oil

2 cloves garlic, peeled and minced

water, enough for desired consistency

3 Tbs. chopped fresh cilantro

PREPARATION TIME: 45 MINUTES

1. To cook either grain, place 2 cups grain in 4 cups water and bring to a boil. Then lower heat, cover, and simmer (15 minutes for quinoa or 30 minutes for brown rice), checking near the end to make sure that all water is absorbed. Turn off heat and let sit for 10 to 15 minutes.

2. Heat 1 Tbs. coconut oil in a large-sized sauté pan over medium heat. Add tofu and brown turning cubes gently. Remove from heat and set aside in a separate bowl.

3. Heat remaining 1 Tbs. oil. Add garlic, carrots, and onion. Stir-fry for 3 to 4 minutes.

4. Add broccoli and stir-fry for another 3 to 4 minutes.

5. Add cabbage, bell peppers, green onions, snow peas and stir-fry for another 2 to 3 minutes.

6. To serve: Place 1 to 2 cups vegetable mixture over 3/4 to 1 cup grain. Spoon tofu over vegetables and sprinkle with sesame seeds. Garnish with cilantro. Serve with Thai Peanut Sauce on the side.

7. *Thai Peanut Sauce:* Place all ingredients except water and cilantro in a 2-cup bowl and mix with a fork. Process until smooth, adding water or orange juice to achieve desired consistency. Add seasonings to taste, adding more tamari for saltiness or more orange juice for sweetness. Let sit for 1 hour before serving. Sprinkle with cilantro just before serving.

Serves 6 to 8

Tofu Cacciatore

This sauce is flavoursome and chock full of vegetables. An excellent way to enjoy tofu. Serve on its own or over whole-grain noodles. Can be made ahead of time and reheated later.

1 lb. firm tofu, cut into smaller-than-dice-sized squares

2 Tbs. olive oil or ghee

2 cloves garlic, crushed

1 cup diced leeks or onions

1 cup diced carrot

1 cup diced celery

3 cups sliced mushrooms

1/2 cup finely chopped fresh basil or 1 tsp. dried basil

2 Tbs. fresh oregano or 1 tsp. dried oregano

3 bay leaves

2 cups tomato sauce (homemade would be excellent)

1 tsp. salt

1 red pepper, diced

1 green pepper, diced

1/2 cup finely chopped fresh parsley

PREPARATION TIME: 30 MINUTES

1. Heat 2 Tbs. oil in a wok and sauté tofu until brown on all sides. Remove from pan.
2. Add remaining oil and cook garlic and leek or onion over medium heat until soft.
3. Add carrot, celery, mushrooms, basil, oregano, bay leaves, and tomato sauce. Cook for 15 to 30 minutes.
4. Add salt, tofu, red and green peppers, and parsley. Cook for 5 minutes until heated through. Remove bay leaves. Adjust salt.

Serves 6 to 8

Vegetarian Stew

Excellent fall and winter fare – vary the vegetables according to availability. Wonderful the next day in a thermos.

2 Tbs. olive oil or ghee

1 medium onion, chopped

1 leek, sliced and washed carefully to remove sand (or use another small onion)

1 cup sliced cabbage, or 1 1/2 cups halved brussel sprouts

10 medium mushrooms, quartered

1 large clove garlic, finely chopped

3 Tbs. spelt flour or whole wheat flour

2 cups (or more)water

2 medium carrots, halved and sliced diagonally

4 medium potatoes, diced

optional vegetables:
corn cobs, halved, brussel sprouts yams, etc.

one 14-ounce can diced tomatoes

one 19-ounce can black beans

1 small can lima beans (optional)

1 Tbs. dry parsley

2 bay leaves

1 tsp. herbes de Provence
(or 1/4 tsp. each thyme, basil, marjoram, and oregano) – or a combination of herbs from your garden

3 Tbs. tamari

salt and pepper, to taste

PREPARATION TIME: 30 MINUTES

1. Fry onion, leek, cabbage, mushrooms, and garlic in oil on medium for 5 to 10 minutes, stirring frequently, until vegetables are soft and golden.
2. Stir in flour until vegetables are coated, and then slowly add water until thickened stirring continuously.
3. Add the rest of the ingredients (except salt and pepper), plus just enough water to cover by 3/4 inch (2 cm.) and simmer for 1 hour until vegetables are tender. Season with salt and pepper, and/or additional tamari. Alternatively, bake this stew in a 375F oven for 1 1/2 hours, removing cover for the last 1/2 hour.

Serves 8 to 10

White Bean Sauce for Pasta

A simple, satisfying make-ahead sauce for any kind of pasta shape. Try it over brown rice or kamut pasta for a change. Thankfully, there are some excellent whole grain pasta alternatives available now.

3/4 cup dry cannellini beans
   (white kidney beans) – or one
   19-ounce can cannellini beans, drained

2 Tbs. olive oil

4 large cloves garlic, finely chopped

3 ribs celery, very finely chopped

1 large ripe tomato (1/2 pound),
   cut into 3/4 inch (2 cm.) cubes

1 tsp. dried basil or 3 Tbs. fresh basil,
   chopped

1/2 cup finely chopped fresh parsley

salt (optional)

pepper

1. To reconstitute beans, soak in enough water to cover by 4 inches (10 cm.), overnight or for at least 8 hours. Drain and rinse thoroughly and place in a pot with enough water to cover by 2 inches (5 cm.). Bring to a boil and then turn heat down and simmer for 1 to 1 1/2 hours, until beans are tender.

2. Heat oil in a large skillet or wok. Add garlic and celery and cook until celery is tender (approximately 10 minutes).

3. Add beans, tomato, basil, parsley, salt, and pepper. Cook for another 5 minutes, until slightly thickened.

4. Serve over hot pasta – rotini, bow ties, ziti, etc.

5. Garnish with freshly grated parmesan, if desired.

Serves 4

"Correcting oneself is correcting the whole world.
The Sun is simply bright.
It does not correct anyone.
Because it shines, the whole world is full of light.
Transforming yourself is a means of giving light to the whole world."

RAMANA MAHARSHI

Raw Main Dishes

Angel Hair with Marinara Sauce

A live food alternative to spaghetti and tomato sauce. A crowd pleaser. To make the angel hair with zucchini, use a spiral slicer which can be purchased at some Asian stores or through my web-site www.carolinedupont.com. Or, simply use a vegetable peeler to create long ribbons

ANGEL HAIR:

2 medium-sized zucchinis

MARINARA:

2 plum tomatoes or 1 whole tomato

10 sun dried tomato halves, soaked for at least 2 hours

1 apple, cored

1/2 red pepper, coarsely chopped

1 clove garlic, chopped

1 1/2 Tbs. lemon juice

2 dates, pitted and soaked for at least 2 hours then chopped

Celtic sea salt, to taste

2 Tbs. olive oil

1/4 cup fresh basil + a few basil leaves set aside and sliced into ribbons for decoration

1 Tbs. fresh oregano or 1/2 tsp. dried oregano

GARNISH SUGGESTIONS:

whole olives

basil ribbons

pine nuts, ground in a coffee grinder, or Pine Nut Parmesan

fresh tomatoes

sun-dried tomatoes, chopped

marinated portabello mushrooms, chopped

PREPARATION TIME: 30 MINUTES

1. Make the angel hair by processing the zucchini in a spiral slicer (or peel with a vegetable peeler to get ribbons – keep turning zucchini to make strands fairly thin). Put angel hair in a large shallow serving bowl. Cut with kitchen scissors or a knife (otherwise some of the noodles could be 10 feet long!)

2. Place marinara ingredients, except herbs, in a blender or food processor and combine until smooth. Add herbs and process for a few more seconds.

3. Taste and adjust seasoning.

4. Wait until just before serving to assemble dish (otherwise marinara will draw water out of zucchini). Toss angel hair with marinara and garnish as desired. Serve immediately.

Serves 4 to 6

MANY OF THE SALADS IN THE RAW SALAD SECTION ARE HEARTY ENOUGH FOR A MEAL, SO CHECK THEM OUT FOR MEAL IDEAS AS WELL. THIS RECIPE AND THE FOLLOWING ONES ARE RAW VERSIONS OF FAVOURITE COOKED MEALS THAT ARE HEALTHY, LIGHT, NOURISHING, AND TASTY.

Ezekiel 4:9 Wraps Ⓛ Ⓢ Ⓓ Ⓣ

Food For Life makes brilliant, delicious, and highly nutritious wraps that have become a staple in our house for quick meals. Although not raw, they are made from living sprouted grains and legumes and cooked without oils at low heat. They are high in protein and the sprouting process makes them digestible and less likely to cause problems for people with wheat and gluten sensitivities. You can find them in the freezer section of your health food store. The following are some of the raw stuffing ideas we have enjoyed with these wraps. Fill centre of wrap, roll, and enjoy!

CLASSIC WRAP:

My kids like this with a little Nasoya mayonnaise spread on the wrap.

lettuce (romaine, leaf, or baby greens)

avocado

cucumber spears

tomatoes

sunflower sprouts and/or red clover (or alfalfa) sprouts

sauerkraut

ASIAN WRAP:

Spread almond butter on the wrap and then add:

baby bok choy

grated carrots

cucumber spears

any kind of sprout

slivered green onions

chopped cilantro

Sprinkle with a little cold pressed sesame oil, and nama shoyu or tamari or salt.

MEXICAN WRAP:

Spread guacamole on the wrap and then add:

sliced lettuce

chopped tomatoes or salsa

chopped green onion

sprouts

chopped cilantro

MIDDLE EASTERN WRAP:

Spread wrap with hummus and add:

tomatoes

cucumbers

sprouts

chopped parsley

shredded lettuce

olives

SALAD STUFFED WRAPS:

Many of the salads in this book are delicious in wraps (for example: 4 F Salad, Kale Avocado Salad, Chinese Cabbage Salad).

SWEET WRAP:

Spread wrap with raw almond butter or organic peanut butter

Add chopped bananas and a drizzle of honey

Indian Curry Salad Meal Ⓛ Ⓖ Ⓓ Ⓣ

This is a complete meal made from raw ingredients. The dressing is mysterious and interesting with its layers of flavours.

DRESSING:

1/3 cup olive oil

1/3 cup lemon juice

1/2 medium avocado

1/4 cup water

2 to 3 Tbs. raw honey or maple syrup
  or 3 large soaked dates

2 tsp. turmeric

2 Tbs. fresh parsley

2 Tbs. cilantro

1 large clove garlic

1 inch (2 1/2 cm.) piece ginger,
  peeled and diced small

1 tsp. Celtic sea salt

1 hot chili pepper or hot sauce (to taste)

SUGGESTED SALAD INGREDIENTS:

3 cups romaine lettuce hearts, sliced

1 1/2 cups diced celery hearts

1 cup sliced arugula

1 1/2 cups sunflower greens

1 cup finely diced broccoli

1/2 small red onion,
  sliced in thin half-moons

2 pickling cucumbers, cut on bias –
  or 1/3 English cucumber, diced

1 small yellow summer squash,
  cut on bias

3/4 cup cubed fresh pineapple

1/2 cup raw cashews

2 to 3 Tbs. currants

2 to 3 Tbs. grated dried coconut

1. Blend dressing ingredients in a blender for approximately 1 minute, until smooth. Taste and adjust seasoning.
2. Place salad ingredients in a large salad bowl. Pour 1 to 2 cups of dressing over vegetables and toss. Serve with remaining dressing on the side. Dressing will keep in the refrigerator for 1 week.

Serves 4 to 6

Pad Thai Ⓛ Ⓖ Ⓓ Ⓣ

Eating a living food diet and craving noodles? Try this adaptation of a Live Café classic.
A spiral slicer is helpful but not mandatory.

VEGETABLE OPTIONS:

zucchini, carrot, red onion, red pepper,
   yellow pepper, red cabbage,
   green apple, cauliflower, coconut
   – about 6 cups total

For example:

2 medium zucchinis, julienned or made
   into noodles in the spiral slicer

1 large carrot, julienned or made into
   noodles in the spiral slicer

1/2 cup thinly sliced red onion,
   or green onion

1/2 red and 1/2 yellow pepper,
   thinly sliced

1 cup slivered red cabbage

1 green apple, julienned

3/4 cup finely chopped cauliflower

3 Tbs. grated coconut

ALMOND CHILI SAUCE:

3 Tbs. maple syrup

1 lemon, juiced (about 2 to 3 Tbs.)

2 small cloves garlic

4 dates, soaked for approximately 2 hours

4 Tbs. nama shoyu or tamari

1 inch (2 1/2 cm.) ginger,
   peeled and chopped

1 tsp. salt

1/4 tsp. cayenne

1/2 cup raw almond butter

1/2 cup water (for thinning)

1. Chop vegetables into a large shallow serving bowl. 'Julienne' means to slice into matchstick sizes.
2. Blend sauce ingredients until smooth. Pour over vegetables just before serving, toss, and enjoy.

Serves 4

Pizza-Raw Ⓛ Ⓖ Ⓓ

CRUST:

Living Buckwheat crusts—
   or Ezekiel 4:9 wraps from the freezer
   section of your health food store, cut
   into 4 and baked at 200F until crisp

CHEESE:

1/2 cup raw almonds, soaked for 4 hours

1/2 cup raw cashews, soaked for 4 hours

1/4 cup lemon juice

1 tsp. Celtic sea salt

1 tsp. garlic

PIZZA SAUCE:

1 cup chopped fresh tomatoes

1/4 cup sun-dried tomatoes (soaked for
   1 to 2 hours if they are very dry)

1/4 cup fresh basil

1/4 cup red pepper

1/2 apple

1 Tbs. fresh oregano or 1/2 tsp. dried

1 tsp. Celtic sea salt

2 Tbs. olive oil

1 Tbs. sweet onion

SUGGESTED GARNISHES:

fresh chopped tomatoes

marinated mushrooms (sliced, marinated
   for 2 to 4 hours in nama shoyu,
   olive oil, and rosemary)

sun-dried tomatoes, chopped

olives (green or black), chopped

fresh herbs: basil ribbons, chopped
   tarragon, rosemary, oregano

red peppers or yellow peppers,
   finely chopped

PREPARATION TIME: 30 MINUTES

1. *Cheese:* Blend until smooth (I find
that using a hand blender is ideal).
Keeps 2 to 3 days in fridge.

2. *Pizza Sauce:* Blend all ingredients
until smooth.

3. Assemble individual pizzas by
spreading cheese on crust, then layering
with sauce and finally garnishes.

Makes 12 four-inch pizzas

Raw Art on a Plate Ⓛ Ⓖ Ⓓ Ⓣ

When I went to do the 9-day third initiation for Kriya Yoga at the Quebec ashram, I was following a completely live foods diet. I was aware that the chef was going to prepare a mostly macrobiotics menu, so I came supplied with much of my own food. To my enjoyment, Dominique, the chef, seemed to delight in making me beautiful salad plates. Every meal was a colourful surprise that he would pull out of the refrigerator with a sparkle in his eye—with an assortment of fresh vegetables, some carved, some chopped, some sliced, some grated, and always a few flowers. When I returned home, I discovered that my children also enjoyed these meals. Some of the appeal is because the infinite designs you can create are delightful to the eye, and these meals take very little time to prepare. I like the fact that, unlike tossed salads, the ingredients stay separate and can be enjoyed in their pure form.

INGREDIENT SUGGESTIONS:

1/2 avocado (can stuff with sauerkraut
or ketchup à la raw)

carrot and/or beet, grated

Carrot-Beet Salad

peppers, sliced

raw pâté (possibly stuffed into a
pepper half or into a few mushrooms)

sprouts (sunflower, buckwheat, clover,
onion, etc.)

red and/or green cabbage, grated

zucchini, grated or sliced

cherry tomatoes

tomatoes, sliced or quartered

radishes, carved

celery sticks

green beans, yellow beans

olives

sauerkraut

walnut halves, pecan halves

fresh herbs

a sprinkling of sunflower seeds, pumpkin
seeds, hemp seeds, sesame seeds

fruit slices, berries

1. Start by laying several lettuce leaves on each plate.
2. Then arrange any of the ingredients in any way that feels appealing to you. It's fun to create designs by varying the shapes and colours of the vegetables and/or fruit. I like to keep the various ingredients relatively separate – anyone can combine them as they please.
3. Top with any dressing (oil and lemon juice or balsamic vinegar works fine too).

Raw Tomato Sauce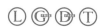

A fresh sauce to make in the late summer/early fall when tomatoes are at their best. My favourite end of summer meal consists of tossing this sauce with raw zucchini noodles made with the spiral slicer. Then I sit on my hammock with the last rays of the day warming me and enjoy.

4 large fresh ripe tomatoes
  (approximately 2 lb.)

1 large clove garlic, minced

4 Tbs. chopped fresh basil

1/2 tsp. salt, to taste

2 Tbs. olive oil

2 Tbs. pine nuts, whole or
  coarsely chopped

2 to 3 zucchinis, sliced into noodles
  with spiral slicer (or very coarsely
  grated or made into ribbons with a
  vegetable peeler) (if using spiral slicer,
  cut noodles with a knife or kitchen
  scissors to make them shorter) – or
  3/4 lb. whole-grain fettucini or
  spaghetti (rice, wheat, or kamut),
  cooked according to package directions,
  drained in a colander and rinsed
  with cool water.

Cheese (optional choices):
  bocconcini, cubed
  feta, crumbled
  parmesan, grated

1. Dice tomatoes. Place in a large shallow serving bowl with garlic, basil, salt, and olive oil.

2. Ideally, let mixture sit at room temperature for 1 hour.

3. Toss tomato mixture with raw or cooked noodles.

4. Add cheese if desired. Serve and enjoy.

Serves 4 to 6

Stir-free ⓁⒼⒹⓉ

A completely raw version of an Oriental favourite. Scrumptious and fresh. Here is an example of a raw foods dish that has all of the 6 essential flavours to fill our senses and our souls. Sweet peppers, carrots, and honey; sour orange and lime juice; bitter cabbage and coriander; astringent broccoli and cauliflower; pungent garlic and ginger; salty shoyu — these are some of the ingredients whose role is partly to fill our need for these flavours. The result is a fully nourishing and satisfying meal.

VEGETABLE IDEAS:

2 cups chopped broccoli and/or
  cauliflower (chopped medium-fine)

1 to 2 ribs celery, sliced on diagonal

1 carrot, sliced in half and
  then sliced on diagonal

3 Tbs. finely sliced sweet Vidalia onion

1/2 cup fresh shitake mushrooms,
  halved and sliced

1/2 red pepper or yellow pepper
  (or a combination), thinly sliced

1 small green zucchini or yellow
  zucchini, halved and thinly sliced

1/2 cup very finely sliced green
  cabbage or red cabbage

1/2 cup quartered and sliced radish
  (daikon, red, or China Rose)

3/4 cup cubed pineapple or mango

1/2 cup raw whole cashews or
  chopped almonds (optional)

1/2 to 1 cup chopped fresh coriander

DRESSING:

1/2 cup fresh squeezed orange juice
  (approximately 1 orange)

1 Tbs. rice vinegar or lemon juice

1 Tbs. grated fresh ginger

1 clove garlic, minced

2 Tbs. nama shoyu or tamari

2 Tbs. cold pressed sesame oil

1 Tbs. sesame seeds (white or black)

1 Tbs. maple or agave syrup or honey

1. Assemble dressing ingredients in
the bottom of a large salad bowl.
Add vegetables, fruit, nuts, coriander.
2. Taste and adjust seasoning.

Serves 4 as a meal, 8 as a side dish

Sushi ⓁⒼⒹ

Instead of rice, layer the carrot almond paté on nori sheets, followed by thinly sliced veggies.
Don't forget to serve this sushi with the traditional fixings: tamari, wasabi and pickled ginger.

nori sheets

CARROT ALMOND PÂTÉ:

1 medium carrot

1 medium parsnip or another carrot

3/4 cup almonds, soaked for 4 to 8 hours

2 Tbs. lemon juice

1 green onion, finely chopped

1 Tbs. dulse powder (optional)

VEGGIES:

sprouts (alfalfa, clover, or
    sunflower work well)

cucumber, julienned

avocado

zucchini, grated

sun-dried tomatoes, soaked and chopped

pineapple, finely cubed

CONDIMENTS:

wasabi

pickled ginger

tamari or nama shoyu

PREPARATION TIME: 30 MINUTES

1. Process carrots, parsnip, and almonds through a masticating juicer or a food processor to create a pâté. Add remaining ingredients for Carrot almond pâté. Taste and adjust accordingly.

2. Spread a couple of spoonfuls of pâté on the nori sheet, leaving approximately 3/4 inch (2 cm.) at the edges closest and farthest from you.

3. Place a small amount of veggies/condiments in a line close to the bottom of the sheet.

4. Using a sushi mat or by hand, roll the sushi from the bottom edge, being careful to keep it even and tight. Moisten the edge of the nori to seal. Lay it on the sealed edge.

5. When ready to serve, cut each roll into 3/4 inch (2 cm.) pieces with a serrated knife (keep knife wet for easier cutting) and serve with wasabi, ginger and nama shoyu or tamari.

6. Nori becomes softer as you let these sit.

Serves 4 to 8

Walnut Burgers Ⓛ Ⓖ Ⓓ

These tasty burgers are completely raw and delicious served on a romaine lettuce leaf with Ketchup A La Raw, sliced tomato, thinly sliced onion, and Marinated Portabello Mushrooms

4 cups walnuts (or pecans),
  soaked for 2 hours

1 1/2 cups carrots, finely chopped

1/4 cup fresh onion (red or sweet),
  divided

1 1/2 cups portabello mushrooms

2 small cloves garlic

1/2 red pepper, finely chopped

8 sun-dried tomato halves, soaked for
  2 hours and finely chopped

1/2 cup fresh parsley, finely chopped
  (or 2 Tbs. dried parsley)

1/4 cup fresh basil, finely chopped
  (or 1 Tbs. dried basil)

1/2 tsp. dried oregano

1/2 Tbs. paprika

1 Tbs. nama shoyu or tamari

1 tsp. Celtic sea salt, to taste

PREPARATION TIME: 30 MINUTES+

1. Blend walnuts, carrots, half the onions, mushrooms, and garlic in a food processor until smooth – or run through a homogenizing juicer using the blank blade. Add all other ingredients and mix well to combine. Taste and adjust seasoning.

2. Form into patties and dehydrate for 2 to 4 hours at 110F. They are tasty without dehydrating but the burgers will be soft. Alternatively, you could put them in an oven at the lowest possible setting for approximately 1 hour.

3. Serve on a romaine lettuce leaf and add raw ketchup (see recipe in Dressings and Sauces section), sliced tomato, thinly sliced onion rings, and Marinated Portabello Mushrooms (see recipe in Vegetables section).

Makes 10 to 12 patties

"Time and again we are queried on our sources of protein.
Where, we ask in return, do the cows, elephants and rhinoceros —
all sturdy, strong creatures — get their protein needs supplied?
From grass, from foliage, from green things, is the answer.
They do not eat refined, cooked, pickled, dehydrated, pasteurized, spiced,
salted, canned, or otherwise conditioned materials.
They are simple creatures eating nature's way.
We try to be the same: simple-living people surviving on simple food,
home grown, organically grown, and simply prepared.
Our foods are vital, nutritional and economical.
For fifty years we have thrived on such
and plan to continue so until our last days."

SCOTT AND HELEN NEARING, *THE GOOD LIFE*,
WHICH DESCRIBES THEIR 60 YEARS OF SELF-SUFFICIENT LIVING

Vegetables

Vegetable Ideas

We often eat our vegetables raw and/or steamed, eaten plain or with a little olive oil or butter. Here are some ideas for variety:

BEETS

Cook until tender, slip skins off, slice, and toss with balsamic vinegar.

BROCCOLI

Steam and then toss with garlic, olive oil, and tamari.

BRUSSELS SPROUTS

Steam until tender, and then toss with a little olive oil and lemon juice.

CARROTS

Slice diagonally, steam, and toss with honey or maple syrup and butter.

CAULIFLOWER

Steam and serve with Cheesy Sauce (see recipe in Dressings and Sauces section).

GREEN BEANS

Steam and toss with chopped almonds, sunflower seeds or pumpkin seeds, drop of tamari, and a little sesame oil.

SQUASH (BUTTERNUT, ACORN, ETC.)

Cut squash in half, scoop out seeds and place face down on a baking dish in about 1/2 inch (1 cm.) of water. Bake at 350F until tender (30 to 45 minutes), scoop out flesh, and mash with sucanat, fresh nutmeg, and butter or coconut butter.

SPAGHETTI SQUASH

Bake squash at 350F until tender (30 to 45 minutes), until strands separate easily. Scoop out flesh and serve topped with any kind of pasta sauce.

ZUCCHINI OR EGGPLANT

Slice large summer zucchini 1/2 inch (1 cm.) thick, brush with olive oil and garlic, and grill. For eggplant, sprinkle with salt first and then absorb bitter juices with a clean tea towel.

Baked Vegetables ⒼⒹⓉ⁺

I have made variations of this dish dozens or maybe hundreds of times. Use vegetables that you have on-hand. When it's red pepper season I will add more of them. This is good on its own but you can also serve it over steamed quinoa, millet, or brown rice.

---

6 to 8 cups vegetables, diced –
some suggestions are:
  1 cup leek and/or onion
  1 to 2 cups mushrooms
  (button, brown, or portabello)
  3 to 4 cups green and/or
  yellow zucchini
  1 cup (or more) red peppers or
  other coloured peppers
  cauliflower
  eggplant

---

garlic, chopped

---

dried herbs or fresh herbs (try a large
  pinch of oregano and basil, or also
  add thyme)

---

1 to 2 Tbs. tamari

---

1 to 2 Tbs. olive oil

---

1 tsp. balsamic vinegar (optional)

---

feta cheese, preferably raw
  (goat's or sheep's) (optional)

---

1. Place the vegetables in a large casserole dish with a lid and toss with garlic, herbs, tamari, oil, and vinegar (if desired).

2. Bake at 350F for 40 minutes until vegetables are tender. Toss in optional feta, put lid back on and let sit for 5 minutes before serving.

TO COOK GRAINS:

Place 1 1/2 cups of grain and 3 cups of water in a medium-sized pot. Bring to a boil, turn down heat to low-medium, cover, and simmer (20 minutes for quinoa, or 30 minutes for brown rice, or 40 minutes for millet). Turn off heat and let sit for 10 minutes.

Serves 4 to 6

Good Greens!

Some greens, particularly mature kale, collards, and mustard greens, can be covered in water to boil rather than stir-fry, to make them less bitter, more tender, and more digestible. However, if the greens are young and the palate is accustomed to the bitterness of greens, you might be inclined to simply add the greens to the frying pan after the leeks or onions are soft. Add a little water and steam until tender. Gomasio is a mixture of salt and ground sesame seeds that can be sprinkled on any vegetables. Make it yourself by grinding 4 Tbs. of sesame seeds with 1 tsp. salt in a coffee grinder and storing in a small shaker jar.

1 bunch Swiss chard, kale, collards, mustard greens, or spinach

Onions or leek and/or garlic, to taste (suggested combination: 1 small onion + 1 leek + 2 cloves garlic)

1 to 2 tsp. cold pressed coconut oil or olive oil or sesame oil

salt or tamari (to season to taste)

Gomasio

1. Gently stir-fry onion and garlic in any cold pressed oil (1 to 2 tsp.) until tender, adding water as necessary to prevent sticking.

2. For mature greens or people new to greens: remove tough stems from the greens and then wash by swishing them around in a sink full of cold water. Coarsely shred, place in a pot, and cover with water. Bring to a boil, turn down heat, and simmer for 5 to 20 minutes depending on the type of greens (spinach takes the least amount of time, collards the most). Make sure you cook the greens until they are tender. Drain thoroughly and add to pan with onion and garlic.

3. For younger greens and experienced green-eaters: wash greens and shred coarsely, leaving some of the stem, as desired. Add to pan raw with a little water once the leeks or onions are soft. Stir, cover with a lid, and allow to steam until tender.

4. Taste, season, and serve. Sprinkle with Gomasio, to individual taste.

Serves 4

Marinated Portabello Mushrooms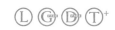

These are such a tasty addition to any meal. You can make them in a dehydrator or an oven.

3 portabello mushrooms, halved and sliced 1/4 inch (1/2 cm.) thick

2 Tbs. olive oil

1 Tbs. fresh lemon juice

1 Tbs. nama shoyu or tamari

1 small clove garlic, minced (optional)

1 Tbs. crushed fresh rosemary

1/2 cup water

1. Mix wet ingredients in the bottom of a glass dish. Add mushrooms and toss gently to coat.

2. Place in dehydrator for 2 to 3 hours at 115F, or bake at 325F for 30 to 40 minutes; mixing at least once to coat mushrooms with sauce.

Makes 3 cups

Mashed Yams

A simple and tasty way to enjoy yams.

4 cups peeled yams, cut into large chunks (3 medium yams)

1 clove garlic, left whole

1 Tbs. honey or maple syrup or agave syrup

1 Tbs. butter or coconut butter

pinch salt

1. Gently steam yam and garlic in 3/4 inch (2 cm.) of water in a medium-sized pot, until tender, about 15 minutes.

2. Drain the water and add salt, sweetener, and butter.

3. Make into a smooth puree using a hand blender or potato masher.

4. Taste and adjust seasoning.

Serves 3 or 4

Root Fries Ⓖ Ⓓ Ⓣ⁺

These colourful and tasty fries are delicious just as they are, but some people might want to dip them in natural ketchup. One of my kids' favourite meals is these fries topped with grated cheese and Tamari Cream Gravy for poutine. This is a great way to introduce root vegetables to your family.

8 cups root vegetables, a combination of:
  potatoes (white, gold, red, and blue)
  yams
  beets
  carrots
  parsnips
  butternut squash
  rutabagas

1 cup sliced leeks or onions and/or
  whole clove garlic (optional)

2 Tbs. ghee (clarified butter) or
  olive oil (or a combination)

Celtic Sea salt, to taste

optional herbs (to taste, try 1/2 tsp.):
  rosemary
  basil
  thyme
  sage

1. Scrub vegetables well, leave peel on and cut into fry shape (many kitchen gadgets can do this, but you can also do it by hand)
2. While preheating the oven to 375F, melt the ghee on a cookie sheet or roasting pan. Add prepared vegetables and toss, adding salt and herbs until coated.
3. Return tray to oven and bake for 30 to 40 minutes, depending on desired crispness.

Serves 4 to 6

Scalloped Potatoes

A very respectable dairy-free version of a favourite.

1 cup raw cashews
4 cups water, divided
1 Tbs. nutritional yeast
2 Tbs. celery
1 Tbs. onion
1 tsp. (or to taste) salt
1 Tbs. + 1 tsp. arrowroot powder
8 medium-large potatoes, peeled and thinly sliced
1 onion, finely chopped

PREPARATION TIME: 30 MINUTES

1. Blend cashews and 1 cup water in blender for 1 minute, until creamy. Make sure there are no cashew pieces left.
2. Add 1 1/2 cups water and remaining ingredients except potatoes and onions, but including the first tablespoon of onion.
3. Pour into saucepan and add remaining 1 1/2 water. Bring to a boil over medium heat, stirring constantly until thickened.
4. In a large casserole dish, alternate layers of sauce, potatoes, and onions, (3 layers), beginning and ending with sauce.
5. Cover with lid or foil. Bake at 350F for 1 hour and 30 minutes. Remove cover halfway through the baking time.

Serves 6 to 8

Don't go outside your house to see the flowers.
My friend, don't bother with that excursion.
Inside your body there are flowers.
One flower has a thousand petals.
That will do for a place to sit.
Sitting there you will have a glimpse of beauty
Inside the body and out of it,
Before gardens and after gardens.

KABIR

Desserts and Treats

Cooked Desserts and Treats:

Apple Crisp
Carob-Cashew Cookies
Coconut-Oatmeal Cookies
Festive Popcorn
Fruit and Nut Bars
Fudgy Multigrain Cookies
Lemon-Date Bars
Peach-Blueberry Crisp
Peanut Butter Spice Cookies
Pecan Pie
Six-Minute Chocolate Cake
Yogourt Cheese Pie

Raw Desserts and Treats:

Apple Raisin Cookies
Banana Cream Pie
Caramel Sauce
Carob Pudding
Cashew Cream
Creamy Lemon Tarts
Living Date Squares
Nut and Seed Bars
Orange-Nutmeg Dream Cake
Pecan-Fig Bars
Shannon's Chocolate Mousse Pie
Truffles
Yam Pie

Apple Crisp ⊤⁺

Apple Crisp is a Canadian classic and most people prefer it over apple pie. Here is a low-fat version without refined sugar.

apples or pears, peeled and sliced

1 cup apple juice

3 Tbs. sucanat

2 Tbs. whole wheat flour or spelt flour

1/4 cup honey or maple syrup

1/4 cup softened butter or coconut butter

1/4 cup water

1/2 tsp. salt

1 tsp. cinnamon

1 tsp. vanilla

2 1/2 cups rolled oats

1/2 cup spelt flour or
   whole wheat pastry flour

1/2 cup chopped nuts (walnuts, pecans,
   or almonds) (optional)

1. Place apples or pears into an 8 inch x 8 inch baking dish until it is 3/4 full.

2. Pour in juice and sprinkle sucanat and flour over fruit, tossing to combine.

3. Whisk together honey, butter, water, salt, cinnamon, and vanilla. Add oats, flour, and optional nuts. Toss until well mixed. Sprinkle this topping over apples.

4. Bake at 350F for 45 minutes or until golden brown.

5. Serve with cashew cream, if desired.

Serves 4 to 6

Carob-Cashew Cookies

These cookies are the creation of my friend and colleague Ricki Heller. She's expert at creating delicious baked goods with whole foods ingredients. She also sells her baked goods at the Village Market in Thornhill on Saturday mornings (and other places), and teaches vegetarian cooking, baking, and nutrition classes. You can find out about her and her services at www.rickiskitchen.com.

1/4 cup pure maple syrup

1/4 cup brown rice syrup

1 tsp. pure vanilla extract

1/4 cup organic sunflower or
other light-tasting oil

1 Tbs. ground flax seed

1/2 tsp. ground cardamom (optional)

1 1/2 cups whole spelt flour

1/4 cup carob powder, sifted

1/2 cup lightly toasted cashews,
finely chopped

1 tsp. baking powder

1/4 tsp. baking soda

PREPARATION TIME: 30 MINUTES

1. Preheat oven to 350F. Lightly grease 2 cookie sheets (or line with parchment paper).
2. In a large bowl, mix together the maple syrup, brown rice syrup, vanilla, oil, flax seed, and cardamom. Whisk to combine (or mix with a fork). Set aside for at least 2 minutes.
3. Meanwhile, combine the flour, carob powder, cashews, baking powder, and baking soda. Pour over the wet ingredients and stir well to combine (the dough should be fairly stiff).
4. Drop the dough by tablespoonfuls onto prepared cookie sheets. Flatten slightly with the back of the spoon or the palm of your hand.
5. Bake in preheated oven for 8 to 10 minutes, until edges begin to brown. Remove from oven and cool completely before removing from sheets. May be frozen.

Makes approximately 20 cookies

Coconut-Oatmeal Cookies

These rich little treats are made with whole foods ingredients.

2/3 cup coconut butter or butter

1 1/4 cups sucanat

1 Tbs. ground flax seed

1 1/4 cup spelt flour

1 cup rolled oats

3/4 cup dried coconut

1 tsp. baking powder

1 tsp. baking soda

1 1/2 cups raisins

PREPARATION TIME: 30 MINUTES

1. Cream butter and sucanat together thoroughly.
2. In a separate bowl combine flax seeds, flour, oats, coconut, baking powder, and baking soda.
3. Add dry ingredients to butter mixture and mix well. Stir in raisins.
4. Drop by spoonfuls onto lightly greased baking sheets. Flatten slightly with a floured fork.
5. Bake at 350F for 10 to 13 minutes, until light golden.

Makes approximately 24 cookies

Festive Popcorn

Yummy!

4 cups air-popped organic popping corn

2 Tbs. butter or coconut butter

1 1/2 tsp. vanilla extract

2 to 3 Tbs. honey

1 Tbs. molasses

1 Tbs. cinnamon

1. In a saucepan over low heat stir together butter, vanilla, honey, and molasses until completely melted. Add cinnamon.
2. Pour over popcorn, tossing to cover kernels.
3. Serve in individual bowls.

Makes 4 cups

Fruit and Nut Bars

There are infinite variations to these healthy treats — use different types of cereal flakes, nut butters, nuts, rolled grains, seeds, and dried fruit.

1/4 cup brown rice syrup or
  barley malt syrup

1/4 cup honey

2 Tbs. coconut butter

1/4 cup raw nut butter (almond, cashew,
  or organic peanut butter)

1 cup cereal flakes
  (any whole-grain flake: multigrain,
  millet, kamut, buckwheat, etc.)

1 cup rolled grains (oats, kamut, or spelt)
  – or for gluten-free version,
  omit and add more buckwheat or
  millet cereal flakes

3/4 cup dried fruit (raisins, chopped
  dates, apricots, dried cranberries,
  blueberries, or cherries)

3/4 cup coarsely chopped raw nuts and
  seeds- any combination (almonds,
  cashews, sunflower seeds,
  pumpkin seeds

1. Gently heat syrup, honey, coconut butter, and nut butter in a large-sized saucepan until melted.
2. Stir in remaining ingredients and then pat into an 8 inch x 8 inch pan.
3. Refrigerate at least 1 hour and then cut into squares or bars.

Makes 10 to 20 bars, depending on size

Fudgy Multigrain Cookies

Great cookies!

1 cup quick oats

2/3 cup spelt flour or whole wheat flour

1/3 cup hemp flour or barley flour or
soy flour

1/2 tsp. baking soda

1/2 tsp. salt

1/3 cup nut butter (peanut, cashew,
soy, or almond)

2 Tbs. soft butter or coconut oil

1 cup sucanat

1/2 cup milk (soy, almond, or dairy)

2 tsp. vanilla extract

2/3 cup semi-sweet chocolate chips or
carob chips

1/3 cup coarsely chopped walnuts

PREPARATION TIME: 30 MINUTES

1. Preheat oven to 325F. Grease several
large baking sheets.
2. In a large bowl, mix oats, flours,
baking soda, and salt.
3. In a small bowl, mix nut butter
and butter until well blended. Stir in
sucanat, milk, and vanilla until combined.
4. Add wet to dry ingredients and stir
with a wooden spoon just until combined.
Gently fold in chocolate chips or carob
chips and walnuts. For tender cookies,
don't overmix the dough.
5. Drop dough by large spoonfuls onto
prepared baking sheets, spacing 2 inches
(5 cm.) apart. Bake 13 to 15 minutes,
until set and tops look dry. Let cool on
baking sheets for 5 minutes before
removing to wire racks to cool completely.

Makes 16 cookies

Lemon-Date Bars

A lovely fresh version of date squares.

2 cups chopped pitted dates

juice of 1 lemon

1/2 cup water

1/2 cup butter or coconut butter

1/2 cup sucanat

1 3/4 cups whole wheat flour or
   light spelt flour

1 tsp. salt

1/2 tsp. baking soda

1 cup rolled oats

PREPARATION TIME: 30 MINUTES

1. Preheat oven to 350F.

2. In a saucepan, combine the dates, lemon juice, and water. Cook, covered, on low heat for 10 minutes stirring occasionally. Remove from heat and set aside.

3. In a bowl, cream together the butter and sucanat. Stir in the flour, salt, and baking soda. Add the oats and mix well using your hands. The dough will be crumbly but will hold together when squeezed.

4. Press 2/3 of the dough into an oiled 8- or 9-inch square baking pan. Stir the date mixture and spread it over the dough. Crumble the remaining dough on top.

5. Bake for 30 minutes. Cool in the pan and cut into bars.

Makes 16 bars

Peach-Blueberry Crisp

Awesome at the end of summer when peaches and blueberries are both in season.

6 cups sliced fresh peeled peaches

2 cups blueberries

1/4 cup sucanat

2 Tbs. whole wheat flour

3 tsp. cinnamon, divided

1 cup oats

1/4 cup maple syrup

4 Tbs. soft organic butter

PREPARATION TIME: 30 MINUTES

1. To peel peaches, pour boiling water over fruit in a bowl, let sit, and rinse under cold water. Peel will remove easily.

2. In an 8-cup baking dish, combine sliced peaches and blueberries. Sprinkle sucanat, flour, and 2 tsp. cinnamon over top and toss to mix.

3. Combine rolled oats, syrup, and remaining cinnamon. Cut in butter until crumbly. Sprinkle over fruit.

4. Bake at 350F for 25 minutes.

Serves 6 to 8

"In the infinity of life where I am, all is perfect whole and complete. I am one with the Power that created me. I am totally receptive to the abundant flow of prosperity that the Universe offers. All my needs and desires are met before I even ask. I am Divinely guided and protected. My good comes from everywhere and everyone. All is well in my world." LOUISE L. HAY

Peanut Butter Spice Cookies

This is another one of Ricki Heller's delicious whole foods baked creations
(www.rickiskitchen.com).

3/4 cup organic peanut butter

1/2 cup soft tofu or silken tofu

1/4 cup organic sunflower oil or olive oil

1 cup sucanat

3 cups whole spelt flour

1 1/2 tsp. baking soda

1 tsp. cinnamon

1/2 tsp. nutmeg

1/4 tsp. allspice

1/2 tsp. ginger

1/2 cup whole oats

3/4 cup organic raisins

PREPARATION TIME: 30 MINUTES

1. Preheat oven to 350F. Lightly grease 2 cookie sheets (or line with parchment paper).
2. In the bowl of a food processor or medium bowl, combine the peanut butter, tofu, oil, and sucanat until smooth and no traces of tofu are visible. Set aside.
3. In a large bowl, sift together the flour, soda, and spices. Mix in the oats and raisins and stir to combine.
4. Pour the wet ingredients over the dry and mix well (it will be a fairly stiff dough).
5. Drop by tablespoonfuls onto cookie sheets and flatten slightly with the back of the spoon or the palm of your hand.
6. Bake for 8 to 10 minutes, until just golden. Allow to cool before removing from sheet.
7. May be frozen.

Makes approximately 30 cookies

Pecan Pie ⓓ

My neighbour and good friend Evelyne made this with sliced almonds instead of pecans and it was a real hit. Be sure to use barley malt syrup, it makes the filling gooey.

DOUGH:

1 1/2 cups light spelt flour or
  whole wheat pastry flour

1/2 tsp. fine sea salt

1/2 cup + 1 Tbs. high oleic safflower oil
  or palm oil shortening or coconut oil

3 1/2 Tbs. water

FILLING:

1/2 cup maple syrup

1/4 cup barley malt syrup
  (buy at health food store)

1/2 tsp. ground cinnamon

1 Tbs. arrowroot powder

2 Tbs. tahini

2 1/2 cups pecan halves or sliced almonds

PREPARATION TIME: 40 MINUTES

1. Preheat oven to 350F.
2. Put the flour and salt in a bowl and stir together. Add the oil and water and stir until it forms a crumbly meal. Gather up into a ball (dough will be moist). Press the dough evenly and firmly into the bottom and up the sides of a 9- or 10-inch pie plate. Use a knife to even out edges. Prick holes into the bottom and sides of the pie shell and bake for 10 to 15 minutes, until light golden.
3. Put the maple syrup, barley malt syrup, cinnamon, arrowroot, and tahini in a food processor and process until smooth. Add the nuts (reserve a handful for decorating) and pulse several preparation times to coarsely chop the nuts.
4. Pour the filling into the baked pie shell and decorate with reserved nuts. Bake until the filling is bubbly and the top is evenly browned (20 to 30 minutes).
5. Cool completely before serving.

Serves 8

246 *cooked desserts and treats*

Six-Minute Chocolate Cake

A fast and delicious chocolate treat — mix it right in the pan. Serve the glaze suggested below or top with your favourite frosting, cashew cream, ice cream, raspberry sauce, or strawberry sauce. See if you can find organic cocoa and chocolate squares — most health food stores will carry them.

1 1/2 cups light spelt flour

1/3 cup cocoa powder
 (preferably organic)

1 tsp. baking soda

1/2 tsp. salt

1 cup sucanat

1/2 cup good quality vegetable oil
 (high oleic safflower is good)

1 cup cold water

1 Tbs. coffee substitute (Bambu, Inca)
 (optional)

2 tsp. pure vanilla extract

2 Tbs. vinegar
 (apple cider vinegar is fine)

GLAZE:

6 squares semi-sweet chocolate
 (6 ounces) (preferably organic)

2/3 cup hot water or soy milk or
 rice milk or dairy milk

1/2 tsp. pure vanilla extract

1. Preheat oven to 375F.
2. Mix together flour, cocoa, baking soda, salt, and sucanat in an ungreased 8-inch square or 9-inch round baking pan.
3. In a 2-cup measuring cup, measure and mix together the oil, water, coffee substitute, and vanilla.
4. Pour the liquid ingredients into the baking pan and mix batter with a fork or small whisk.
5. When the batter is smooth, add the vinegar and stir quickly. There will be pale swirls in the batter where the baking soda and the vinegar are reacting. Stir just until the vinegar is evenly distributed throughout the batter.
6. Bake for 25 to 30 minutes. Set cake aside to cool.
7. To make the glaze, reset the oven to 300F. Melt the chocolate in a small ovenproof bowl in the oven for about 10 minutes.
8. Stir the hot liquid and the vanilla into the chocolate until smooth.
9. Spoon the glaze over the cooked cake. Refrigerate for at least 30 minutes before serving.

Serves 8

Yogourt Cheese Pie

Try to use one of the excellent organic yogourts currently available for this fresh pie. Saugeen County and Pinehedge Farms are two brands available in Ontario.

1 quart plain natural yogourt
(contains NO gelatin)

1 1/2 tsp. vanilla

1/3 cup maple syrup

1 1/2 cups crushed graham crackers
(buy a sugar-free organic brand at the
health food store)

1/4 cup butter or coconut butter, melted

2 Tbs. sucanat (optional)

2 to 4 cups berries or sliced fruit
(strawberries, peaches, blueberries,
raspberries, pitted cherries)

PREPARATION TIME: 30 MINUTES

1. *The night or morning before you will serve this pie, prepare the Yogourt Cheese:* Line a colander or large sieve with overlapping coffee filters or several layers of cheese-cloth; Place the colander or sieve in a large bowl; Spoon in the yogourt and cover with a plate or plastic wrap; Refrigerate for at least 10 hours; After 3 or 4 hours or overnight, pour out the liquid collected in the bowl and return to fridge; The yogourt will thicken to the consistency of cream cheese; Discard or drink the liquid.

3. Blend vanilla and maple syrup into yogourt cheese by hand.

4. Prepare the pie crust: In an 8- or 9-inch pie pan, mix the graham cracker crumbs with the melted butter and the sucanat; Stir well and press into the pie pan evenly; Spread the yogourt cheese over the crust; Top with the fresh fruit.

5. Serve right away or chill until ready to serve. Alternatively, you can serve the cheese pie plain and then top each individual serving with fruit.

Serves 6 to 8

Apple Raisin Cookies

These delicious little treats are raw and full of life-giving enzymes. To cook them, they are dehydrated in a dehydrator or an oven at low temperatures.

2 cups sunflower seeds,
soaked 6 to 8 hours

2 apples, Fuji works well

2 large bananas

1/2 cup honey dates

1 tsp. vanilla or
2 inches scraped vanilla bean

1 tsp. cinnamon

1 cup raisins

1 cup walnuts, soaked for 6 to 8 hours
and chopped

> THESE GOOD-FOR-YOU RAW
> DESSERTS CAN BE EATEN GUILT-FREE
> ANYTIME. THEY ARE MADE WITH
> WHOLE FOODS ONLY AND MANY CAN
> EVEN BE EATEN AS A MEAL (ESPECIAL-
> LY THE PIES) MAYBE WITH A SALAD.

PREPARATION TIME: 40 MINUTES+

1. Process sunflower seeds, apples, bananas, and dates through a food processor using the S-blade (or a Champion Juicer using the solid plate).
2. In a large bowl, mix dough with vanilla, cinnamon, raisins, and walnuts.
3. If using a dehydrator, spoon dough onto the dehydrator tray with a non-stick sheet and form into small round cookies. If using the oven, place cookies on 2 cookie sheets lined with a teflex sheet or wax paper. Flatten with the back of the spoon.
4. Dehydrate at 105F for 6 to 10 hours, then turn cookies over, remove nonstick sheet, and continue dehydrating for another 2 to 4 hours (or until desired texture is obtained). I like them chewy and slightly moist.
5. If using oven, turn temperature knob until oven just comes on, place cookies in oven and keep door slightly propped open with the handle of a wooden spoon. Cook/dehydrate for 6 to 10 hours, turning cookies over halfway through, until desired dryness is reached (time will depend on heat of oven, try to keep it as low as possible to maintain the enzymatic activity of the raw ingredients).

Makes 36 small cookies

Banana Cream Pie Ⓛ Ⓖ Ⓓ

Another raw desert that's sure to please.

CRUST:

1 1/4 cups raw almonds, soaked for
  4 hours, drained and rinsed

1 cup dates, chopped

1 Tbs. water (as necessary)

1/2 tsp. vanilla (optional)

dash cinnamon or cardamom (optional)

BANANA CREAM:

6 to 8 frozen very ripe bananas
  (prepare by peeling, breaking into
  pieces, and freezing in resealable bags)

1 cup frozen dried coconut

1/2 cup frozen dates, chopped

1 tsp. vanilla

1 to 2 Tbs. (or to taste) maple syrup
  (optional)

2 Tbs. coconut

PREPARATION TIME: 40 MINUTES

1. Dry almonds with a towel. In a food
processor, chop the nuts until they are
ground. Add dates and process until the
mixture is uniform. Add water, vanilla,
and cinnamon and continue processing.
Mixture should hold together – add
water if necessary.

2. Press mixture into an 8- or 9-inch
square or circular pan. Use immediately
or dehydrate in the sun or a warm oven.

3. In a heavy-duty juicer, using the
blank screen, alternate putting bananas,
coconut, and dates through the
machine into a chilled bowl. Quickly
stir in the vanilla and the optional
maple syrup. Pour mixture into crust
smoothing with the back of a spoon.
Top with coconut. (You could also use
a powerful blender like Vitamix or
Blendtech to make the banana cream.
Start with a small amount of bananas,
blend, and gradually add more.)

4. Place in the freezer immediately,
covering with wax paper. Before
serving, let sit in the refrigerator for
15 minutes to soften slightly.

Serves 4 to 6

Caramel Sauce   Ⓛ Ⓖ Ⓓ Ⓣ

This lovely raw sauce goes well on everything.

5 Tbs. almond butter	1. Blend all ingredients until smooth, adding a small amount of water as needed to achieve desired consistency.
1/4 cup maple syrup or agave syrup	
2 Tbs. cold pressed coconut oil	2. Keeps well in the refrigerator.
1 Tbs. vanilla extract	
2 pitted soft dates	Makes 2/3 cup
pinch sea salt	
pinch cinnamon	
raw carob powder or cocoa powder (for a chocolate-y treat) (optional)	

Carob Pudding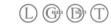

A creamy, sweet, live treat.

1/2 cup raw cashews, soaked for 4 hours and drained	1. Drain and reserve raisin or date soak water. Blend all ingredients together on medium speed for 2 to 3 minutes, gradually adding soak water as needed until pudding is creamy and smooth.
2 ripe bananas	
1/2 cup raisins or dates, soaked for 1 hour	
2 Tbs. carob powder	
1 tsp. vanilla or 2 inches (5 cm.) scraped vanilla bean	Serves 1 or 2
pinch salt	

Cashew Cream Ⓛ Ⓖ Ⓓ Ⓣ

A delicious alternative to ice cream. Serve over fruit crumbles or pies.

1 cup cashews, soaked in water to cover for 4 hours
1 to 1 1/2 cups water
2 Tbs. (or to taste) maple syrup
1 tsp. vanilla or 2 inches (5 cm.) scraped vanilla bean
dash salt (optional)

1. Blend all ingredients together until smooth and creamy. Start with 1 cup of water and add just enough to reach desired consistency.
2. Refrigerate until ready to serve.

Makes 2 cups

Creamy Lemon Tarts Ⓛ Ⓖ Ⓓ

These creamy little delights are simple and a lovely finish to any special meal. Thank you Jennifer Italiano from Live Café in Toronto.

CRUST:

2 cups soaked almonds
6 soaked dates or very soft dates
1 Tbs. maple syrup
1 Tbs. non-alcohol vanilla extract
pinch sea salt

FILLING:

2 cups soaked cashews
1/2 cup lemon juice
1/4 tsp. vanilla
4 soaked dates or very soft dates
2 Tbs. maple syrup or agave syrup

PREPARATION TIME: 40 MINUTES

1. Process crust ingredients in a food processor until mixed. If you prefer a chunky crust, pulse until desired consistency is achieved. For a smoother crust process longer. Place in muffin trays (oil with coconut oil and don't pack too tightly) and dehydrate at 115F for 12 hours (or until firm).
2. Process filling ingredients in a blender until completely smooth. Fill crusts and enjoy.

Makes approximately 12 tarts

Living Date Squares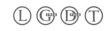

All date square connoisseurs who I served these to raved about them.

FILLING:

2 cups chopped pitted dates

2 Tbs. water

juice of 1 large orange (1/2 to 3/4 cup)

zest of 1 large orange

CRUST:

2 cups pecans or walnuts

1 cup raw oats ground in a
 coffee grinder or oat flour

dash cinnamon

4 Tbs. maple syrup

1. Soak dates in water and juice for 30 to 60 minutes. If you are using soft fresh dates, then you can omit the soaking time and use less orange juice.
2. Coarsely grind nuts in a food processor. Add ground oats or oat flour and pulse to mix.
3. Add cinnamon first, then maple syrup one tablespoon at a time until the mixture holds together.
4. Lightly oil a 9-inch square pan with coconut oil or olive oil.
5. Press a little over half of the crust mixture into the bottom of the pan, reserving the rest for later.
6. Puree the date and orange juice mixture until smooth in a food processor. Spread over the crust.
7. Crumble the remaining half of the crust mixture over the dates and compress with a spoon or your hands.
8. Optional: place in the sun or a dehydrator at 115F for a few hours.

Makes 12 squares

Nut and Seed Bars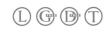

A natural power bar and a good fix when you're craving something sweet and rich. Keep logs in freezer until ready to slice and eat. Vary the nuts and seeds as you like. To entice kids who are reluctant to be adventurous with their food choices, try using an organic peanut butter instead of almond butter.

1 cup almonds or cashews or walnuts (or a combination)

1 cup seeds (sunflower, sesame, pumpkin, hemp, or a combination)

1/2 cup dried unsweetened shredded coconut (optional)

1/2 cup soft dates, pits removed

1/2 cup raisins or more dates

3 Tbs. raw almond butter or

1 Tbs. water (or enough to make mixture stick, may not be needed depending on moistness of dates)

OPTIONAL INGREDIENTS:

4 Tbs. raw carob or cacao powder (grind raw cacao nibs in coffee grinder)

1 to 2 Tbs. spirulina or barley green or other green powder

1 Tbs. maca

1. Grind the nuts, seeds, and coconut to a fine meal in a food processor. Add the fruit, the nut butter, and optional ingredients and process to a ball, adding water only as needed.
2. Roll into 2 to 3 logs, 1 1/4 inch (3 cm.) diameter, wrap in wax paper and then place logs in a plastic bag.
3. Freeze for at least 2 hours.
4. Keep logs frozen and slice into 1/2 inch (1 cm.) thick rounds when desired.

Orange-Nutmeg Dream Cake

Proof that healthy desserts can also be heavenly. You could easily and guiltlessly have this cake as a meal!

2 cups almonds, dry
1 cup pecans, dry
1 1/2 cups dates, soaked pitted
2 Tbs. carob powder
juice of 1 orange (1/2 to 3/4 cup)
1 tsp. vanilla
3/4 to 1 tsp. nutmeg (preferably freshly grated)
5 frozen bananas, thinly sliced if you are using a food processor
1 to 2 tsp. finely grated orange peel
1 large ripe mango
maple syrup, to taste (optional)

PREPARATION TIME: 40 MINUTES+

1. In a food processor, grind almonds and pecans (reserve 8 to 10 for decorating). Add dates (reserve 6 for cream) and process until chopped medium-fine. Add carob, orange juice, 1/2 tsp. vanilla, and nutmeg and process in pulses until dough-like but still slightly chunky. Add water or orange juice if necessary to get desired result. Place in a loose-based round cake tin (cover the base with cling wrap and the sides with foil, if desired, for easier removal.)

2. The cream can be made in a homogenizing juicer or a food processor. For the juicer method, use the blank plate and process frozen bananas, mango meat, and remaining dates. Mix in remaining vanilla and orange peel. Taste and add a little maple syrup if desired. In a food processor, process all of the above ingredients, scraping down the sides to make sure that the mixture is fluffy and creamy.

3. Place this on top of the cake mixture in the tin, smoothing out with a spatula, and decorating with pecans and a sprinkling of nutmeg. Return to the freezer for a least 1 hour. Take it out and remove from tin approximately 10 to 15 minutes before serving.

Serves 8 to 12

Pecan-Fig Bars Ⓛ Ⓖ Ⓓ Ⓣ

Another one of Jennifer's brilliant raw desserts.

2 cups pecans

1 cup soaked figs (remove stems), drained (drink the soak water – it's good!)

1 Tbs. vanilla extract (non-alcohol)

ICING:

1/2 cup raisins, soaked for 20 minutes in apple juice

3/4 cup apple juice

1/2 Tbs. cinnamon

1 Tbs. psyllium

1. Soak raisins in apple juice for approximately 20 minutes.
2. Chop pecans in a food processor. Add soaked figs and vanilla. Pat this mixture into an 8- or 9-inch square tray, approximately 1 inch (2 1/2 cm.) thick.
3. Cut into squares. Put in freezer for 15 minutes until set.
4. Meanwhile, blend icing ingredients in a blender until smooth. Let stand in refrigerator for 15 minutes, until firm.
5. Put a dollop of icing on each bar, garnish with a whole pecan, and serve.

Makes 12 to 16 bars

Shannon's Chocolate Mousse Pie

My friend Shannon Harlow is a wonderful vegetarian cook. She made us this pie one evening and unfortunately the first edition of this book was already off to the printer. Here it is now for you to enjoy too!

CRUST:

1 cup raw almonds

3 dates

honey or maple syrup

FILLING:

4 ripe avocadoes

16 soft, fresh dates, pitted

2 heaping Tbs. cocoa powder

3 to 6 Tbs. agave syrup (to taste)

TOPPING:

Fresh berries, or blend them with a little agave syrup if desired

PREPARATION TIME: 40 MINUTES+

1. Grind almonds in a food processor, then add dates and mix until texture is uniform. Add a little honey or maple syrup until mixture sticks together. Press into an 8-inch round pie pan.

2. Cut avocados in half, remove pit and scoop flesh into a food processor. Add dates, cocoa powder and sweetener and blend until completely smooth. Taste and add more sweetener if desired.

3. Pour filling into prepared crust and refrigerate at least a couple of hours.

4. Serve with fresh berries, mashing a little with a fork to form a chunky sauce, adding sweetener if desired.

Serves 6 to 8

Truffles Ⓛ Ⓖ Ⓓ Ⓣ

A sweet ending to any meal.

---

1 1/2 cups walnuts (or use half cashews)

3/4 cup soft dates

2 to 4 Tbs. raw carob powder or raw
  cacao nibs ground in a coffee grinder

1 to 3 Tbs. water or orange juice, as
  needed (depends on moistness of dates)

1/2 cup chopped dried apricots or
  dried coconut or orange rind or
  other dried fruit (optional)

1. Grind the nuts into a fine meal in food processor.

2. Add dates and process until smooth.

3. Mix in carob powder and chosen liquid if needed (so that mixture sticks).

4. Mix in optional fruit if desired.

5. Roll into small balls and then roll in carob or coconut if desired.

Makes 18 to 24 truffles

Yam Pie Ⓛ Ⓖ Ⓓ

This wonderful raw pie is adapted from Nomi Shannon's excellent cookbook The Raw Gourmet. It's one of my favourites in the fall and winter. Ideally this should be made with a powerful blender such as Vitamix or Blendtech.

PREPARATION TIME: 40 MINUTES+

CRUST:

1 1/4 cups almonds, soaked for 8 to 12 hours

1/2 cup honey dates

1 to 1 1/2 Tbs. water

FILLING:

3/4 cup dates, soaked for 20 minutes, drained and then pitted and coarsely chopped (omit soaking if dates are very soft)

1/4 cup raisins, soaked for 20 minutes and drained

3 to 6 yams (depending on size, enough to make at least 4 cups pureed), peeled and cut into chunks

1 tsp. cinnamon

1 tsp. vanilla or 1 to 2 inches (2 1/2 to 5 cm.) vanilla bean, scraped

1/4 tsp. allspice

pinch cloves

pinch nutmeg

pinch sea salt

2 Tbs. psyllium

1. Drain almonds and dry with a clean tea towel. In a food processor, chop the nuts until finely and evenly ground. Add the dates and process until they are evenly incorporated and finely ground. Add enough water for the crust to hold together. Press the mixture into an 8- or 9-inch pie plate. If desired you can dehydrate the crust in a warm oven or the sun or a dehydrator for up to 1 hour.

2. In a food processor, process dates, raisins, and yams until very smooth. Gradually add the spices. At this point, if the filling is not smooth enough, transfer to a blender and blend until smooth, using a spatula to move the mixture down into the blade. Then gradually add the psyllium with the machine running. Pour the filling into the crust and refrigerate for at least 1 hour.

3. Serve topped with Cashew Cream.

Serves 6 to 8

"...forget not that the earth delights to feel your bare feet
and the winds long to play with your hair."

KAHLIL GIBRAN

Appendix

Soaking and Sprouting

Soaking and sprouting optimizes the nutrient value, digestibility, and life force of nuts, seeds, grains, and legumes.

Instructions for soaking

1. Fill a glass or ceramic container no more than 1/2 full with nuts, seeds, or grains.

2. Fill the container with purified water.

3. Soaking time will vary. Refer to individual recipes.

4. After soaking, discard water and rinse thoroughly several times. Soaked nuts, seeds, or grains can be stored in fresh water in the refrigerator for 2 to 3 days. If the nuts, seeds, or grains are going to be sprouted, refer to the sprouting process outlined below.

Instructions for sprouting

1. Use soaked nuts, seeds, or grains prepared according to instructions above.

2. Drain and place in a glass jar with a fine mesh screen secured over the top with a rubber band. (This keeps out insects and allows for aeration.)

3. Place nuts, seeds, or grains in a dark area for 24 hours and then expose to indirect sunlight.

4. Sprouts should be rinsed 1 to 2 times a day (more often in warm weather) by filling the jar with water, swishing, and draining with the screen in place – repeat twice. For proper drainage, jar should be stored upside down at a 50- to 70-degree angle. Prop in a bowl or dish rack.

5. When the sprouts reach their specified length, store them in the refrigerator to slow their growth and preserve their freshness.

Reconstituting Dried Beans

1. Use half the amount of dry beans as are needed in the recipe. For example, if 2 cups beans are needed in a recipe, use 1 cup dry.

2. Rinse beans in a strainer, discarding stones and odd looking beans.

3. Soak beans for at least 8 hours in a bowl on the counter. Cover with about 2 inches (5 cm of water).

4. Drain and rinse beans several times in a colander.

5. Add beans and enough water to cover by 2 inches to a good-sized pot.

6. Bring to a boil, reduce heat and simmer until ready.

7. Beans are ready when they are very soft. Cooking time varies according to the type of bean and the age of the bean. Generally they take 30 minutes to 2 hours.

8. Try not to mix different batches of the same type of bean because they often cook at different rates. So if a recipe is calling for 2 cups of dry beans and you have 2 1/2 cups left, finish them off and then restock the next time you are shopping.

9. *To decrease gassiness caused by beans:*
   a. Start with small amounts.
   b. Make sure they are well cooked.
   c. Chew them well.
   d. Combine them with vegetables only.
   e. Add a strip of kombu to the cooking water.

Glossary

You will find all of these ingredients at your local health food store or in the natural foods section of your grocery store.

AGAVE SYRUP
Liquid sweetener made from a cactus. Has a low glycemic index and is considered raw. Unlike honey and maple syrup, it doesn't have a distinctive flavour.

ARROWROOT
Starch flour used for thickening, less processed than cornstarch.

BALSAMIC VINEGAR
A red-brown Italian vinegar made from grapes aged in wooden barrels. Has a rich sweet-sour taste.

CELTIC SEA SALT
A grey unrefined sea salt with a lovely depth of flavour.

MISO
A salty paste made from cooked aged beans and/or grains. Used for flavouring and soup bases.

NAMA SHOYU
A raw version of tamari or soya sauce.

NUTRITIONAL YEAST
A good tasting yeast that adds a cheesy flavour to recipes. Sometimes called Engevita yeast.

SUCANAT
Granulated sugar cane juice. Retains all nutrients except fiber and water. Use 1-to-1 for sugar.

TAHINI
A thick smooth paste made of ground, raw, or toasted sesame seeds.

TAMARI

A naturally brewed soya sauce that contains no sugar or preservatives.

TEMPEH

Fermented soybeans.Probably the healthiest way to enjoy soy, because the fermentation makes it easier to digest. It is usually perpared cubed and flavoured.

TOFU

Soya bean curd, high in protein. Japanese tofu, or silken tofu, has a smoother consistency and can be used in sauces, puddings, dressings, and baked goods. A common brand name is Mori-Nu. Chinese tofu is usually firmer and denser and lends itself well to stir-frys, imitation cottage or feta cheese, and sandwich spreads (Soy City, La Soyarie, and Sol Cuisine are good brands).

Index

A

B

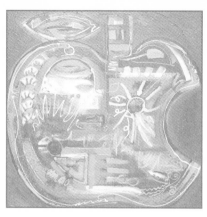

Cover Art: Apple Series #8, 48″x48″, 2005
by Césan d'Ornellas Levine

Enlightened Art: Nourishment for the Spirit

Our deepest and highest selves are nourished first by our thoughts, which in turn influence, and are influenced by, what we choose to ingest and surround ourselves with. Good food, beautiful architecture, art, natural objects… Our spirit responds to the super sensuous world expressed as taste, smell, sound, texture, color, form, and line. Depending on the intention behind them, these choices can serve to either harden and rigidify us or support flow and the shedding of light into our own perfect places of inspirational newness.

My earliest inspirational influence was a group of Algonkin shamans, who created the petroglyphs over a thousand years ago near Peterborough, Ontario, where I grew up in the sixties. My parents took me there often in my childhood to hike and lounge on a limestone slab into which were carved hundreds of images depicting soul retrievals and an ancient animistic cosmology. Running my fingers over those carvings was my first experience of art, and simultaneously, my first experience of the numinous. This treasure trove, known locally as 'the teaching rocks', are now housed in a government building to protect them from being touched and the elements.

Later, as an adult, I discovered my deepest inspiration in the paintings and writings of Wassily Kandinsky. The artist, he argued, has a responsibility to carefully tend the soul through self-development—through awareness of actions, thoughts and feelings. Spiritual discipline is the anchor to which one can tether art making, so the muses themselves have the opportunity to deconstruct the image, and let color, line and texture carry the 'inner note' of a perceptible immanence. This connection between a way of living and the authentic power of the work as something other than 'art for art's sake' resonates deeply for me.

The iconography, approach and technique of my painting arise from a life long immersion in the study of creativity itself, and the maintenance of expanded states of consciousness through the making of art, yoga, meditation and attention to diet. Caroline Dupont's work has been an excellent resource and inspiration.

Césan

Césan exhibits and sells her work internationally through galleries, special venues, private collectors and by commission. Her studio/residence is in Richmond Hill, Ontario, Canada. Online Gallery: www.cesan.ca   Enquiries: info@cesan.ca

Pray to your Heavenly Father:

"Our Father which art in heaven, hallowed be thy name.
Thy kingdom come.
Thy will be done on earth as it is in heaven.
Give us this day our daily bread.
And forgive us our debts, as we forgive our debtors.
And lead us not into temptation, but deliver us from evil.
For thine is the kingdom, the power, and the glory, for ever.
Amen."

Pray to your Earthly Mother:

"Our Mother which art upon earth, hallowed be thy name.
Thy kingdom come,
Thy will be done in us, as it is in thee.
As thou sendest every day thy angels, send them to us also.
Forgive us our sins, as we atone all our sins against thee.
And lead us not into sickness, but deliver us from all evil.
For thine is the earth, the body, and the health.
Amen."

FROM THE ESSENE GOSPEL OF PEACE
TRANSLATED BY EDMUND BORDEAUX SZEKELY

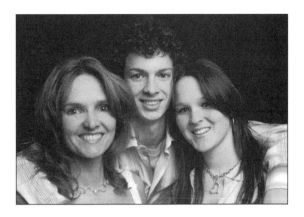

About the Author

Caroline has been inspired and drawn to the field of human health and personal growth as long as she can remember. Her path has led her to the study of fitness and movement, nutrition, the human energy field, yoga and meditation, the art of balanced living and becoming our authentic selves. She holds a Master's degree in Exercise Physiology, a black Belt in the Nia Technique (a holistic fitness approach), is a registered holistic nutritionist, a certified yoga instructor and has attained personal mastery in Reiki Tummo. She is the author of the book *Enlightened Eating* and the CD *Open Heart Meditation*. Through her company Health and Beyond, she works with clients individually as a Holistic Health Practitioner, focusing on Energy Work, Assisted Meditation, One-on-One Yoga, and nutrition, teaches yoga, meditation, whole and living foods preparation, and presents on various health-related topics. She teaches for the Canadian School of Natural Nutrition and lives in Richmond Hill, Ontario with her two children.

Visit her online at www.carolinedupont.com.

See these and other fine raw foods books from the publishers of Enlightened Eating

To find your favorite vegetarian and soyfood products online, visit:

www.healthy-eating.com

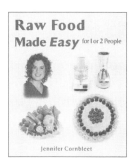

Raw Food Made Easy
Jennifer Cornbleet
978-1-57067-175-3 $16.95

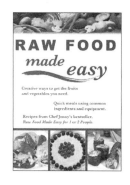

**Raw Food Made Easy
DVD**
Jennifer Cornbleet
978-1-57067-203-3 $19.95

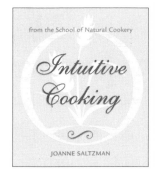

Intuitive Cooking
Joanne Saltzman
978-1-57067-194-4 $19.95

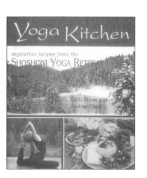

Yoga Kitchen
Faith Stone, Rachael Guidry
978-1-57067-145-6 $18.95

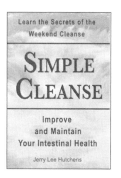

Simple Cleanse
Jerry Lee Hutchens
978-1-57067-172-2 $9.95

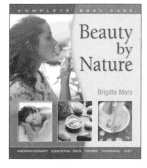

Beauty by Nature
Brigitte Mars
978-1-57067-193-7 $18.95

Purchase these health titles and cookbooks from your local bookstore or natural food store, or you can buy them directly from:

Book Publishing Company • P.O. Box 99 • Summertown, TN 38483 • 1-800-695-2241

Please include $3.95 per book for shipping and handling.